Improving and Equity of Care for People with Serious Illness

PROCEEDINGS OF A WORKSHOP

Laurene Graig, Sylara Marie Cruz, and Joe Alper, *Rapporteurs*

Roundtable on Quality Care for People with Serious Illness

Board on Health Care Services

Board on Health Sciences Policy

Health and Medicine Division

The National Academies of
SCIENCES · ENGINEERING · MEDICINE

THE NATIONAL ACADEMIES PRESS
Washington, DC
www.nap.edu

THE NATIONAL ACADEMIES PRESS   500 Fifth Street, NW   Washington, DC 20001

This activity was supported by Contract No. HHSN263201800029I (Task Order No. 75N98019F00851) with the National Institutes of Health's National Institute of Nursing Research and by Aetna Inc., Altarum Institute, American Academy of Hospice and Palliative Medicine, American Cancer Society, American Geriatrics Society, Anthem Inc., Ascension Health, Association of Professional Chaplains, Association of Rehabilitation Nurses, Blue Cross Blue Shield Association, Blue Cross Blue Shield of Massachusetts, Blue Cross and Blue Shield of North Carolina, Bristol-Myers Squibb, The California State University Shiley Institute for Palliative Care, Cambia Health Solutions, Cedars-Sinai Health System, Center to Advance Palliative Care, Centers for Medicare & Medicaid Services, Coalition to Transform Advanced Care, Excellus BlueCross BlueShield, Federation of American Hospitals, Greenwall Foundation, The John A. Hartford Foundation, Hospice & Palliative Nurses Association, Kaiser Permanente, Susan G. Komen, Gordon and Betty Moore Foundation, National Coalition for Hospice and Palliative Care, National Hospice and Palliative Care Organization, National Palliative Care Research Center, National Patient Advocate Foundation, National Quality Forum, The New York Academy of Medicine, Oncology Nursing Society, Patient-Centered Outcomes Research Institute, Social Work Hospice & Palliative Care Network, Supportive Care Coalition, and the National Academy of Medicine. Any opinions, findings, conclusions, or recommendations expressed in this publication do not necessarily reflect the views of any organization or agency that provided support for the project.

International Standard Book Number-13: 978-0-309-49589-9
International Standard Book Number-10: 0-309-49589-X
Digital Object Identifier: https://doi.org/10.17226/25530

Additional copies of this publication are available from the National Academies Press, 500 Fifth Street, NW, Keck 360, Washington, DC 20001; (800) 624-6242 or (202) 334-3313.

Suggested citation: National Academies of Sciences, Engineering, and Medicine. 2019. *Improving access to and equity of care for people with serious illness: Proceedings of a workshop.* Washington, DC: The National Academies Press. https://doi.org/10.17226/25530.

The National Academies of
SCIENCES · ENGINEERING · MEDICINE

The **National Academy of Sciences** was established in 1863 by an Act of Congress, signed by President Lincoln, as a private, nongovernmental institution to advise the nation on issues related to science and technology. Members are elected by their peers for outstanding contributions to research. Dr. Marcia McNutt is president.

The **National Academy of Engineering** was established in 1964 under the charter of the National Academy of Sciences to bring the practices of engineering to advising the nation. Members are elected by their peers for extraordinary contributions to engineering. Dr. John L. Anderson is president.

The **National Academy of Medicine** (formerly the Institute of Medicine) was established in 1970 under the charter of the National Academy of Sciences to advise the nation on medical and health issues. Members are elected by their peers for distinguished contributions to medicine and health. Dr. Victor J. Dzau is president.

The three Academies work together as the **National Academies of Sciences, Engineering, and Medicine** to provide independent, objective analysis and advice to the nation and conduct other activities to solve complex problems and inform public policy decisions. The National Academies also encourage education and research, recognize outstanding contributions to knowledge, and increase public understanding in matters of science, engineering, and medicine.

Learn more about the National Academies of Sciences, Engineering, and Medicine at **www.nationalacademies.org**.

The National Academies of
SCIENCES · ENGINEERING · MEDICINE

Consensus Study Reports published by the National Academies of Sciences, Engineering, and Medicine document the evidence-based consensus on the study's statement of task by an authoring committee of experts. Reports typically include findings, conclusions, and recommendations based on information gathered by the committee and the committee's deliberations. Each report has been subjected to a rigorous and independent peer-review process and it represents the position of the National Academies on the statement of task.

Proceedings published by the National Academies of Sciences, Engineering, and Medicine chronicle the presentations and discussions at a workshop, symposium, or other event convened by the National Academies. The statements and opinions contained in proceedings are those of the participants and are not endorsed by other participants, the planning committee, or the National Academies.

For information about other products and activities of the National Academies, please visit www.nationalacademies.org/about/whatwedo.

PLANNING COMMITTEE FOR A WORKSHOP ON IMPROVING ACCESS TO AND EQUITY OF CARE FOR PEOPLE WITH SERIOUS ILLNESS[1]

DARCI GRAVES (*Co-Chair*), Special Assistant to the Director, Office of Minority Health, Centers for Medicare & Medicaid Services

PEGGY MAGUIRE (*Co-Chair*), President and Board Chair, Cambia Health Foundation

KIMBERLY D. ACQUAVIVA, Professor, The George Washington University School of Nursing

ROBERT A. BERGAMINI, Medical Director, Palliative Care Services, Mercy Clinic Children's Cancer and Hematology, representing the Supportive Care Coalition

SHONTA CHAMBERS, Executive Vice President of Health Equity Initiatives and Community Engagement, Patient Advocate Foundation

MARSHALL CHIN, Richard Parrillo Family Professor of Healthcare Ethics, Department of Medicine, The University of Chicago Pritzker School of Medicine

ZIAD R. HAYDAR, Senior Vice President and Chief Clinical Officer, Ascension Health

HAIDEN HUSKAMP, 30th Anniversary Professor of Health Care Policy, Harvard Medical School

KIMBERLY JOHNSON, Associate Professor of Medicine, Senior Fellow in the Center for the Study of Aging and Human Development, Duke University School of Medicine

DIANE E. MEIER, Director, Center to Advance Palliative Care

THOMAS M. PRISELAC, President and Chief Executive Officer, Cedars-Sinai Health System

JOANNE REIFSNYDER, Executive Vice President, Clinical Operations and Chief Nursing Officer, Genesis Healthcare, representing the Hospice & Palliative Nurses Association

---

[1] The National Academies of Sciences, Engineering, and Medicine's planning committees are solely responsible for organizing the workshop, identifying topics, and choosing speakers. The responsibility for the published Proceedings of a Workshop rests with the workshop rapporteurs and the institution.

SUSAN ELIZABETH WANG, Regional Lead for Shared Decision-Making and Advance Care Planning, Southern California Permanente Medical Group, Kaiser Permanente

Project Staff

LAURENE GRAIG, Director, Roundtable on Quality Care for People with Serious Illness
SYLARA MARIE CRUZ, Research Associate (*until October 2019*)
RAJBIR KAUR, Senior Program Assistant (*until October 2019*)
SHARYL NASS, Director, Board on Health Care Services, and Director, National Cancer Policy Forum
INDIA OLCHEFSKE, Research Associate (*until June 2019*)
ANDREW M. POPE, Director, Board on Health Sciences Policy

Consultant

JOE ALPER, Consulting Writer

ROUNDTABLE ON QUALITY CARE
FOR PEOPLE WITH SERIOUS ILLNESS[1]

LEONARD D. SCHAEFFER (*Chair*), Judge Robert Maclay Widney Chair and Professor, University of Southern California

JAMES A. TULSKY (*Vice Chair*), Chair, Department of Psychosocial Oncology and Palliative Care, Dana-Farber Cancer Institute; Chief, Division of Palliative Medicine, Brigham and Women's Hospital; Professor of Medicine and Co-Director, Center for Palliative Care, Harvard Medical School

JENNIFER BALLENTINE, Executive Director, California State University Institute for Palliative Care

ROBERT A. BERGAMINI, Medical Director, Palliative Care Services, Mercy Clinic Children's Cancer and Hematology, representing the Supportive Care Coalition

LORI BISHOP, Vice President of Palliative and Advanced Care, National Hospice and Palliative Care Organization

PATRICIA A. BOMBA, Vice President and Medical Director, Geriatrics, Excellus BlueCross BlueShield

SUSAN BROWN, Senior Director, Health Education, Susan G. Komen

GRACE B. CAMPBELL, Assistant Professor, Department of Acute and Tertiary Care, University of Pittsburgh School of Nursing, representing the Association of Rehabilitation Nurses

JANE CARMODY, Program Officer, The John A. Hartford Foundation

STEVEN CLAUSER, Director, Healthcare Delivery and Disparities Research Program, Patient-Centered Outcomes Research Institute

DAVID J. DEBONO, National Medical Director for Oncology, Anthem Inc.

CHRISTOPHER M. DEZII, Lead, Quality and Measure Development, State and Federal Payment Agencies, U.S. Value, Access and Payment, Bristol-Myers Squibb

ANDREW DREYFUS, President and Chief Executive Officer, Blue Cross Blue Shield of Massachusetts

---

[1] The National Academies of Sciences, Engineering, and Medicine's forums and round-tables do not issue, review, or approve individual documents. The responsibility for the published Proceedings of a Workshop rests with the workshop rapporteurs and the institution.

CAROLE REDDING FLAMM, Executive Medical Director, Blue Cross Blue Shield Association

MARK B. GANZ, President and Chief Executive Officer, Cambia Health Solutions

ZIAD R. HAYDAR, Senior Vice President and Chief Clinical Officer, Ascension Health

PAMELA S. HINDS, Director of Nursing Research and Quality Outcomes, Children's National Health System

HAIDEN HUSKAMP, 30th Anniversary Professor of Health Care Policy, Harvard Medical School

KIMBERLY JOHNSON, Associate Professor of Medicine, Senior Fellow in the Center for the Study of Aging and Human Development, Duke University School of Medicine

CHARLES N. KAHN III, President and Chief Executive Officer, Federation of American Hospitals

REBECCA A. KIRCH, Executive Vice President of Healthcare Quality and Value, National Patient Advocate Foundation

TOM KOUTSOUMPAS, Cofounder, Coalition to Transform Advanced Care

SHARI M. LING, Deputy Chief Medical Officer, Centers for Medicare & Medicaid Services

BERNARD LO, President and Chief Executive Officer, Greenwall Foundation

JOANNE LYNN, Director, Center for Elder Care and Advanced Illness, Altarum Institute

DIANE E. MEIER, Director, Center to Advance Palliative Care

AMY MELNICK, Executive Director, National Coalition for Hospice and Palliative Care

JERI L. MILLER, Chief, Office of End-of-Life and Palliative Care Research and Senior Policy Analyst, Division of Extramural Science Programs, National Institute of Nursing Research, National Institutes of Health

R. SEAN MORRISON, Director, National Palliative Care Research Center

BRENDA NEVIDJON, Chief Executive Officer, Oncology Nursing Society

HAROLD L. PAZ, Executive Vice President and Chief Medical Officer, Aetna Inc.

JUDITH R. PERES, Long-term and Palliative Care Consultant, Clinical Social Worker and Board Member, Social Work Hospice & Palliative Care Network

PHILLIP A. PIZZO, Founding Director, Stanford Distinguished Careers Institute; Former Dean, Stanford School of Medicine and David and Susan Heckerman Professor of Pediatrics and of Microbiology and Immunology, Stanford School of Medicine

THOMAS M. PRISELAC, President and Chief Executive Officer, Cedars-Sinai Health System

RAHUL RAJKUMAR, Senior Vice President and Chief Medical Officer, Blue Cross and Blue Shield of North Carolina

JOANNE REIFSNYDER, Executive Vice President, Clinical Operations and Chief Nursing Officer, Genesis Healthcare, representing the Hospice & Palliative Nurses Association

RACHEL ROILAND, Director, Serious Illness Care Initiative, National Quality Forum

JUDITH A. SALERNO, President, The New York Academy of Medicine

DIANE SCHWEITZER, Acting Chief Program Officer, Patient Care Program, Gordon and Betty Moore Foundation

KATRINA M. SCOTT, Oncology Chaplain, Massachusetts General Hospital, representing the Association of Professional Chaplains

KATHERINE SHARPE, Senior Vice President, Patient and Caregiver Support, American Cancer Society

JOSEPH W. SHEGA, Regional Medical Director, VITAS Hospice Care, representing the American Geriatrics Society

CHRISTIAN SINCLAIR, Outpatient Palliative Oncology Lead, Division of Palliative Medicine, University of Kansas Medical Center, representing the American Academy of Hospice and Palliative Medicine

SUSAN ELIZABETH WANG, Regional Lead for Shared Decision-Making and Advance Care Planning, Southern California Permanente Medical Group, Kaiser Permanente

Reviewers

This Proceedings of a Workshop was reviewed in draft form by individuals chosen for their diverse perspectives and technical expertise. The purpose of this independent review is to provide candid and critical comments that will assist the National Academies of Sciences, Engineering, and Medicine in making each published proceedings as sound as possible and to ensure that it meets the institutional standards for quality, objectivity, evidence, and responsiveness to the charge. The review comments and draft manuscript remain confidential to protect the integrity of the process.

We thank the following individuals for their review of this proceedings:

SARAH DOWNER, Health Law and Policy Clinic, Harvard Law School

EDWARD MACHTINGER, Center to Advance Trauma-informed Health Care, University of California, San Francisco

Although the reviewers listed above provided many constructive comments and suggestions, they were not asked to endorse the content of the proceedings, nor did they see the final draft before its release. The review of this proceedings was overseen by **JOHN AYANIAN,** Institute for Healthcare Policy & Innovation, University of Michigan. He was responsible for making certain that an independent examination of this proceedings was carried out in accordance with standards of the National Academies and that all review comments were carefully considered. Responsibility for the final content rests entirely with the rapporteurs and the National Academies.

Acknowledgments

The National Academies of Sciences, Engineering, and Medicine's Roundtable on Quality Care for People with Serious Illness wishes to express its sincere gratitude to the planning committee co-chairs Darci Graves and Peggy Maguire for their valuable contributions to the development and orchestration of this workshop. The roundtable also wishes to thank all of the members of the planning committee, who collaborated to ensure a workshop complete with informative presentations and rich discussions. Finally, the roundtable thanks the speakers and moderators, who generously shared their expertise and their time with workshop participants.

Support from the many annual sponsors of the Roundtable on Quality Care is critical to the roundtable's work. The sponsors include Aetna Inc., Altarum Institute, American Academy of Hospice and Palliative Medicine, American Cancer Society, American Geriatrics Society, Anthem Inc., Ascension Health, Association of Professional Chaplains, Association of Rehabilitation Nurses, Blue Cross Blue Shield Association, Blue Cross Blue Shield of Massachusetts, Blue Cross and Blue Shield of North Carolina, Bristol-Myers Squibb, The California State University Shiley Institute for Palliative Care, Cambia Health Solutions, Cedars-Sinai Health System, Center to Advance Palliative Care, Centers for Medicare & Medicaid Services, Coalition to Transform Advanced Care, Excellus BlueCross BlueShield, Federation of American Hospitals, Greenwall Foundation, The John A. Hartford

Foundation, Hospice & Palliative Nurses Association, Kaiser Permanente, Susan G. Komen, Gordon and Betty Moore Foundation, National Coalition for Hospice and Palliative Care, National Hospice and Palliative Care Organization, National Institute of Nursing Research, National Palliative Care Research Center, National Patient Advocate Foundation, National Quality Forum, The New York Academy of Medicine, Oncology Nursing Society, Patient-Centered Outcomes Research Institute, Social Work Hospice & Palliative Care Network, Supportive Care Coalition, and the National Academy of Medicine.

Contents

Boxes and Figures

Acronyms and Abbreviations

ACA	Patient Protection and Affordable Care Act
ACE	adverse childhood experience
ACP	advance care planning
CACCC	Chinese American Coalition for Compassionate Care
CEP	Community Empowerment Partner
CHW	community health worker
CMS	Centers for Medicare & Medicaid Services
C-TAC	Coalition to Transform Advanced Care
ECANA	Endometrial Cancer Action Network for African-Americans
FPL	federal poverty level
HCBS	home- and community-based services
IOM	Institute of Medicine
LGBT	lesbian, gay, bisexual, and transgender
LTSS	long-term services and supports

NHPCO   National Hospice and Palliative Care Organization
NIH   National Institutes of Health
NP   nurse practitioner
NQF   National Quality Forum

PA   physician assistant
PCORI   Patient-Centered Outcomes Research Institute

RWJF   Robert Wood Johnson Foundation

SFHN   San Francisco Health Network

UCSF   University of California, San Francisco

Proceedings of a Workshop

INTRODUCTION[1]

Millions of people in the United States face the challenge of living with serious illnesses, such as heart and lung disease, cancer, diabetes, and Alzheimer's disease and other forms of dementia. Additionally, many suffer from multiple chronic conditions. According to estimates by the Centers for Disease Control and Prevention,[2] approximately 40 million people have limitations in their usual daily activities as a consequence of serious illness. Providing care to the large and growing portion of the population with serious illness is further complicated by challenges related to inequitable access and disparities in care. These disparities are partly due to, or exacerbated by, factors such as race, ethnicity, gender, geography, socioeconomic status, or insurance status.

The National Academies of Sciences, Engineering, and Medicine's Roundtable on Quality Care for People with Serious Illness hosted a public

---

[1] The planning committee's role was limited to planning the workshop, and the Proceedings of a Workshop was prepared by the workshop rapporteurs as a factual summary of what occurred at the workshop. Statements, recommendations, and opinions expressed are those of individual presenters and participants and are not necessarily endorsed or verified by the National Academies of Sciences, Engineering, and Medicine, and they should not be construed as reflecting any group consensus.

[2] For more information, see https://www.cdc.gov/nchs/data/series/sr_10/sr10_259.pdf (accessed July 17, 2019).

1

workshop, Improving Access to and Equity of Care for People with Serious Illness, with the key objective of exploring the barriers that impede access to care and affect health equity for people with serious illness. On April 4, 2019, in Washington, DC, the workshop highlighted different models of care delivery that serve various communities and vulnerable populations, with the aim of addressing opportunities to minimize barriers, inform policy initiatives, and determine areas for further research in improving access to and equity of care for people with serious illness.

The workshop sessions were developed using the social ecological model (see Figure 1) as a conceptual framework. The social ecological model presents opportunities to understand how stakeholders at various levels throughout the system—including individual, organizational, community, and policy levels—might contribute to advancing access and equity in the care of people with serious illness.

With the social ecological model as a framework:

1. The workshop's first session provided a foundational overview of the challenges and opportunities related to improving access and advancing health equity for people of all ages living with serious illness and explored the role of trauma-informed care.
2. The second session illuminated the opportunities for improving access to and equity of care at the community and organizational levels.
3. The third session explored access and equity from the perspective of patients, families, and clinicians.
4. The fourth session examined policy options to expand access to health care and advance health equity.
5. The workshop concluded with a solutions-focused, moderated discussion of practical next steps to advance health equity and expand access to care for people of all ages living with all stages of serious illness.

Workshop planning committee co-chair Peggy Maguire, president of Cambia Health Foundation, opened the workshop with an overview of the day. In her opinion, disparities in serious illness care are best viewed as social justice issues. According to Maguire, "How we advocate for people with serious illness and their caregivers is a measure of who we are as a country." Therefore, "it requires us to look at these issues through a health equity lens," which "means listening to people that we serve, acknowledging their experiences, and then challenging ourselves to take a hard look at our own

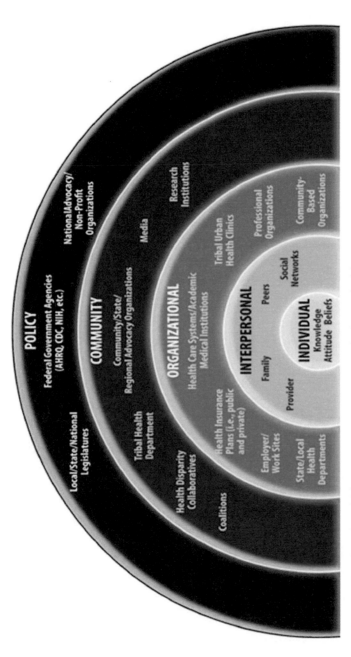

FIGURE 1 A social ecological model for improving access to care and achieving health equity.

NOTE: AHRQ = Agency for Healthcare Research and Quality; CDC = Centers for Disease Control and Prevention; NIH = National Institutes of Health.

SOURCES: As presented by Darci Graves, April 4, 2019; CDC, 2011.

institutions and organizations and how they may perpetuate bias," she said. Maguire concluded her introductory remarks by sharing her hope that the workshop would challenge workshop attendees' thinking about access to and equity of care for people with serious illness. She also hoped the workshop discussions would inspire the attendees to take action to change the status quo so that all people with serious illness have access to high-quality care in the setting that is most appropriate for them.

Darci Graves, workshop planning committee co-chair and special assistant to the director of the Office of Minority Health at the Centers for Medicare & Medicaid Services (CMS), reminded the workshop attendees that equity is one of the six domains of health care quality (safe, effective, timely, equitable, patient-centered, and efficient care) identified by the Institute of Medicine[3] (IOM, 2001). Graves commented that equity is often afforded less attention than other domains: "So, every time we talk about equity today, I want to remind folks that we are talking about a fundamental part of quality." She emphasized that equity is not "extra" or "someone else's department." She asserted that "equity is a fundamental part of quality, and we are all here to improve health care quality." At the same time, no single individual, organization, or policy is going to fix the challenges regarding access and equity in serious illness care. "It is going to take all of us working collaboratively," stated Graves.

The Roundtable on Quality Care for People with Serious Illness serves to convene stakeholders from government, academia, industry, professional associations, nonprofit advocacy groups, and philanthropies. Inspired by and expanding on the work of the IOM's *Dying in America: Improving Quality and Honoring Individual Preferences Near the End of Life* consensus study report (IOM, 2015), the roundtable aims to foster ongoing dialogue about crucial policy and research issues to accelerate and sustain progress in care for people of all ages with serious illness through workshops and other activities.

This Proceedings of a Workshop summarizes the presentations and discussions from the public workshop Improving Access to and Equity of Care for People with Serious Illness. The speakers, panelists, and workshop participants presented a broad range of views and ideas, and Box 1 provides

---

[3] As of March 2016, the Health and Medicine division of the National Academies of Sciences, Engineering, and Medicine continues the consensus studies and convening activities previously carried out by the Institute of Medicine (IOM). The IOM name is used to refer to publications issued prior to July 2015.

BOX 1
Suggestions Made by Individual Workshop Participants for Improving Access to and Equity of Care for People with Serious Illness

Designing and Implementing Programs to Address Inequity
- Design interventions that address equity directly rather than use generic quality improvement interventions. (Chin)
- Address the social determinants of health and payment structures to achieve health equity. (Chin)
- Ensure that any efforts to address health inequities are developed with input from the most severely affected. (Dawes)
- Create or secure funding mechanisms that can sustain innovative, evidence-based, or promising programs that are advancing health equity. (Dawes)
- Use evidence-based solutions to address problems of poor access and inequity that are appropriate for each organization's context. (Chin, Johnson, Maguire)
- Design effective interventions that are multifactorial; are part of culturally tailored quality improvement initiatives; provide nurse-led, team-based care; include families and communities as part of the care team; use community health workers; and provide interactive, skills-based training to patients. (Chin)
- Conduct a root cause analysis that includes those affected by disparities before developing and implementing quality improvement interventions that make equity an integral part of quality. (Chin)
- Implement palliative care consultation in health systems and increase the number of patients who engage in advance care planning to reduce health disparities. (Johnson, Maguire)
- Implement trauma-informed care practices to enable clinicians to meaningfully address the experiences of individual-, family-, and community-level trauma that underlie and perpetuate most health disparities. (Machtinger)
- Address an organization's culture when implementing equity interventions. (Chin, Stokes)
- Build solutions with the voice of the community in mind. (Maguire)

continued

BOX 1 Continued

- Iteratively address specific barriers and facilitators to change based on real-world experience. (Chin)
- Turn to the field of implementation science for help with rolling out a new intervention within health systems. (Chin)
- Frame health equity as a moral and social justice issue. (Chin, Maguire)

Improving Workforce Training and Education
- Commit to achieving health equity by implementing interactional and experiential training on cultural competency and health disparities for health care workers. (Chin)
- Provide incentives for clinicians to participate in training on high-quality serious illness communication. (Sanders)
- Build the capacity of the workforce to understand the role that trauma plays in access, delivery, and adherence. (Dawes)
- Foster a more diverse, team-based approach to serious illness care through education, communication training, and leadership development that includes community health workers. (Maguire)
- Include conversations that acknowledge both the historical and current experiences that most marginalized and vulnerable populations deal with throughout their lives in the training of health care workers. (Barrett)
- Facilitate conversations to achieve care that is consistent with patient preferences. (Johnson)
- Offer more educational opportunities in medical and nursing schools for students to learn about lesbian, gay, bisexual, and transgender (LGBT) health issues. (Margolies)
- Teach health care providers how to advocate for patients who need to address obstacles outside of health care that adversely affect their health. (Chen, Pizzo, Salerno)
- Create culturally appropriate services and education materials so that individuals with little or no English proficiency can communicate effectively with health care providers. (Stokes)
- Provide a pathway to change the culture of health care delivery to one of health equity and to improve the nature of communication and relationships to one where patients feel safe, cared for, and respected through trauma-informed health care. (Machtinger)

BOX 1 Continued

- Ensure health systems support clinicians with communication-related processes that reduce implicit bias, such as Vital Talk. (Sanders)

Developing Partnerships and Including Nontraditional Health Care Workers

- Use an ecological approach, leverage peers, ensure access to high-quality communication, and build partnerships at all levels to address health inequities. (Dawes)
- Improve the care experience and reduce disparities in serious illness care by participating in community education, outreach, and partnerships with the people and institutions in the community with whom patients have their daily interactions outside of the health care system. (Barrett, Francioni, Johnson)
- Include nontraditional workers, such as community health workers, in the health care team to address barriers to equitable care. (Johnson)
- Develop and use community-based partnerships to help break down barriers to access and to extend and deepen the healing available in traditional health care settings. (Machtinger)
- Involve community health workers to serve as cultural bridges between the clinic and community and act as advocates for patients in the clinical setting. (Barrett, Merecias)
- Engage community health workers and places of worship to encourage advance care planning across all populations and develop a trustworthy space for patients in marginalized and underrepresented communities. (Barrett, Maguire)
- Partner effectively with those who are experts in the other areas that contribute to poor access and health inequities, such as housing. (Barrett, Chin)
- Engage and integrate peer navigators into health care to address disparities. (Machtinger)
- Use peer navigators to increase access and achieve health equity, and employ community health workers to educate and improve community health in ways that go beyond their traditional role of care coordinators. (Clauser)

continued

BOX 1 Continued

Pursuing Potential Policy Initiatives and Future Research

- Mobilize individuals to tell their powerful stories to policy makers to drive home the importance of increasing access to care and reducing health inequities. (Clauser, Dawes)
- Design quality of care and payment policies to explicitly achieve health equity. To be effective, those policies should provide adequate resources and support for health equity and quality of care while also holding the system accountable through mandated public monitoring and evaluation. (Chin)
- Focus on developing and implementing actionable and meaningful policies that use an equity lens and accommodate a range of beliefs, values, and concerns. (Dawes)
- Reimagine the U.S. health care enterprise's role in addressing the social determinants of health as if the goal of the enterprise is to keep people healthy rather than treating them when they are sick. (Slavitt)
- Increase eligibility for home- and community-based services offered to Medicaid beneficiaries. (Rowland)
- Expand the home- and community-based benefit to reduce the reliance of many states on the mandatory Medicaid nursing home benefit. (Rowland)
- Cap Medicare Part D catastrophic coverage expenses. (Rowland)
- Restructure the hospice benefit for the seriously ill so that more people get access to holistic care and receive timely and appropriate access to the full benefit when they need it. (Bishop)
- Improve workforce training and consumer education through the Palliative Care and Hospice Education and Training Act. (Bishop)
- Increase access in underserved, rural, and lower economic urban areas through the Rural Access to Hospice Act. (Bishop)
- Financially reward quality and equity in value-based arrangements. (Maguire)
- Improve research on the ways in which health systems exert influence over the awareness of the social determinants of health. (Maguire)

a summary of individual participants' suggestions for potential actions. Appendixes A and B contain the workshop's Statement of Task and workshop agenda, respectively. The workshop speakers' presentations have been archived online (as PDF and audio files).[4]

UNDERSTANDING THE CONTEXT FOR IMPROVING ACCESS TO AND EQUITY OF CARE FOR PEOPLE WITH SERIOUS ILLNESS

The first session provided context for exploring the broader issues of expanding access to care and advancing health equity. It also served to launch the workshop from the individual level of the social ecological model by grounding the discussions in the real-world experience of a person facing the challenges of serious illness.

A Patient's Perspective on Access to and Equity of Care for People with Serious Illness

Bridgette Hempstead, president and founder of Cierra Sisters, opened the workshop's first session with the story of her breast cancer diagnosis in 1996: she was about to turn 35 and went to her physician for a mammogram. She was told that the prevailing guidelines for all women to have a baseline mammogram at age 35 was only for White women because African American women are "not affected by breast cancer." "You have to remember that in 1996, only White women were celebrating breast cancer survivorship," said Hempstead. Fortunately, Hempstead insisted on getting a mammogram, and her physician called on her 35th birthday to inform her that her mammogram indicated that she had breast cancer. Based on her experience, Hempstead founded Cierra Sisters,[5] an advocacy organization with a mission to "break the cycle of fear and increase knowledge concerning breast cancer in the African American and underserved communities" (Cierra Sisters, 2019). "If you have knowledge, you have the power to fight against the effects of breast cancer," said Hempstead.

In 2014, Hempstead was once again diagnosed with cancer, which had metastasized to her lungs and liver. Unfortunately, she said, it did not

---

[4] For more information, see http://nationalacademies.org/hmd/Activities/HealthServices/QualityCareforSeriousIllnessRoundtable/2019-APR-04.aspx (accessed May 23, 2019).

[5] For more information, see http://www.cierrasisters.org (accessed May 21, 2019).

seem like the health care system had improved much for African American women in the 18 years since her first cancer diagnosis. She explained that when she was seen in the hospital emergency department, despite the fact that she was having severe trouble breathing, she was passed from one doctor at the end of a shift to another. In the process, she received unclear orders on what to do next. The first doctor told her that she needed to call her physician the next day to follow up on something unusual on her chest X-ray. In contrast, the second doctor gave her a bottle of cough medicine and told her to come back in a few weeks if her condition did not improve. Fortunately, Hempstead took the first doctor's advice; her physician reviewed her health record and discovered that the second emergency department doctor had erased the first doctor's order, even though the X-rays showed an anomaly that warranted further tests.

In delivering the diagnosis of metastatic breast cancer, Hempstead's oncologist told her that she would not live longer than 1 year and would never sing again, but 6 months later, she sang the national anthem at a Seattle Seahawks football game. By that time, she knew enough about cancer and possible treatments that she was shocked when her oncologist did not offer her the treatment options typically presented to White women; additionally, her oncologist did not refer her for participation in a clinical trial.

Hempstead's response to her unequal treatment by the medical care system was to launch Community Empowerment Partners (CEPs), a program designed to educate women in the African American community about prevention and early detection and provide the skills to navigate the complex health care system. Initially, 14 women recruited from Cierra Sisters received training; these women have since educated more than 120 others within their social networks. Collaborating with investigators at the Fred Hutchinson Cancer Research Center and the University of Illinois at Chicago, Hempstead and colleague Cynthia Green conducted pre- and post-training tests and found that it is feasible to train peer educators to increase knowledge among community members (Hempstead et al., 2018).

Despite the efforts of Cierra Sisters and other advocacy organizations, the health care system is still "broken" for the African American community, in Hempstead's view. "We have to continue to scream at the top of our lungs to make a difference in our community," said Hempstead, "and it should not be like this." Cierra Sisters has now expanded to address inequities in treatment for African American women with endometrial cancer. The resulting Endometrial Cancer Action Network for African-Americans (ECANA) is using the same CEPs model to educate and empower women in the community. In March 2019, ECANA held a national workshop at which representatives from 11 states were trained to be educators in their communities. The goal of all of these efforts, noted Hempstead, is for African American women to receive the same care as White women.

Lessons Learned for Achieving Health Equity Across Diverse Populations

Marshall Chin, the Richard Parrillo Family Professor of Health Care Ethics at The University of Chicago, began his presentation with five lessons he has learned from more than 20 years of work on multi-level interventions to achieve health equity:

1. There is no magic bullet solution to achieving equity in health care.
2. Achieving health equity is a process.
3. Addressing the social determinants of health is essential.
4. Addressing payments and incentives is essential.
5. Equity must be framed as a moral and social justice issue.

The ultimate goal of work in this area, said Chin, should be to improve the national statistics as listed in the Agency for Healthcare Research and Quality's National Healthcare Quality and Disparities reports.[6] "As opposed to a frame of purely improving equity in your own organization, I am talking [about] how do we improve equity nationally, so we move the national numbers," he stressed.

Chin explained that the first lesson grew out of work conducted around 2005 that documented many causes of health disparities while identifying a few overarching solutions for those causes. As the current director of a Robert Wood Johnson Foundation (RWJF) health equity program, Finding Answers: Disparities Research for Change,[7] his belief was that the program would fund grantees, develop solutions, and disseminate them widely. It did not take him long, however, to realize that approach was not going to work due to the importance of context. "You might have a wonderful program for African Americans in Birmingham, Alabama, but that may or may not work for African Americans on the South Side of Chicago," said Chin.

---

[6] For more information, see https://www.ahrq.gov/research/findings/nhqrdr/index.html (accessed May 1, 2019).

[7] For more information, see https://www.solvingdisparities.org (accessed June 26, 2019).

He added that the same holds true for different health care organizations operating in different political and financial contexts. Every health care system, for example, has a different mix of fee-for-service and value-based managed care. An organization's history and the ways in which disparities developed over time can also influence what interventions will work best, according to Chin.

The bottom line, said Chin, is that every organization has to work through its own solutions. He noted that there is still value in having a selection of evidence-based solutions that organizations can use as a starting point to tailor their own interventions. Chin pointed out that his review of more than 400 papers on interventions to address health care disparities did not find many common themes in terms of what works to reduce inequities. However, he was able to identify a few commonalities among effective interventions, including those that were multifactorial; were culturally tailored quality improvement initiatives; had nurse-led, team-based care; integrated family members and community partners; used community health workers; and provided interactive, skill-based training to patients (Chin et al., 2012).

Chin explained there are multiple levels for taking action in both the clinical and policy areas (Chin et al., 2012), and he presented a model for action in which a person lives in the context of the community and its knowledge of health care. For example, Hempstead's African American community had little awareness about breast cancer issues. When she became a patient, she encountered health care providers who lacked communication skills and knowledge of breast cancer in African American women.

In addressing the second lesson—that achieving equity is a process—Chin detailed the key components as outlined by RWJF's Advancing Health Equity: Roadmap for Reducing Disparities (see Box 2).[8]

Chin noted that the third lesson—addressing the social determinants of health—is currently perhaps the most popular issue in the field of health disparities. He explained that most health care organizations are now looking at individual patients, trying to identify their specific needs and referring them to local community-based organizations that can address those needs. Chin's ideal world would have a communication conduit that sends information from the community-based organizations to the health care system. According to Chin, fewer health systems are addressing the underlying structural drivers of health care disparities, such as the structural racism

---

[8] For more information, see https://www.solvingdisparities.org/implement-change/roadmap-reduce-disparities (accessed May 1, 2019).

BOX 2
Advancing Health Equity:
Roadmap for Reducing Disparities

Create a Culture of Equity
- Go beyond cultural competency training and stratifying clinical performance measures by race.
- Interventions with great tactics and strategies for implementation will fail if equity is not a part of an organization's culture.

Implement Quality Improvement Infrastructure and Process
- Situate equity as a cross-cutting dimension that underlies all other dimensions of quality.
- Quality improvement efforts have to start with a root cause analysis that identifies the drivers of disparities.
- Include the community and those affected by disparities who are likely to have a different lived experience than that of health care professionals.

Make Equity an Integral Part of Quality
- Iteratively address specific barriers and facilitators to change.

Design Interventions with an Equity Lens
- Design interventions in a way that they address equity directly.
- Tailor interventions to address the specific situations and drivers of disparities present in a health care organization.

Implement, Evaluate, and Adjust Interventions
- Ask why a proposed intervention will improve the status quo.
- Identify any external incentives, such as different payment models, that can be drivers for the implementation process.
- Identify the culture of the organization and subsequently develop a plan for executing and evaluating the intervention.

Sustain Interventions
- Implementing, evaluating, adjusting, and sustaining interventions are important for long-term success.

SOURCES: As presented by Marshall Chin, April 4, 2019; Chin et al., 2012; Clarke et al., 2012.

that leads to segregated housing and income inequality. What is needed, Chin asserted, are free, frank, and fearless discussions about structural racism, colonialism, social privilege, and intersectoral partnerships to address those underlying structural drivers. Having such discussions can be difficult, according to Chin, at least in part because power differentials influence the historical narrative and control over resources, thus affecting the way in which health disparity issues are framed.

In Chin's view, the fourth lesson—efforts to address payment and incentives—and the social determinants of health are the two frontier areas in the health disparities field. Chin pointed out the large gap between the rhetoric about how the United States values health equity as expressed in documents, such as *Healthy People 2020*, and actual policies that do little to support and incentivize health equity. Instead, he said, the nation needs to explicitly design quality of care and payment policies to achieve health equity. Policies should provide adequate resources and support for such efforts, while also holding the health care system accountable through mandated public monitoring and evaluation.

Chin noted that the National Quality Forum (NQF) published a roadmap for promoting health equity based on what it called the "Four *I*s":

1. Identify priority disparity areas,
2. Implement evidence-based interventions to reduce disparities,
3. Invest in health equity performance measures, and
4. Incentivize the reductions of health disparities and achievement of health equity (NQF, 2017).

Of the 10 recommendations NQF made to incentivize the reduction of health disparities and achievement of health equity, Chin focused on the importance of accountability, redesigning payment models to support health equity, and tailoring the safety net. Accountability, he said, entails stratifying clinical performance measures by factors such as race, ethnicity, socioeconomic status, disability status, and serious illness.

Turning to the newest iteration of his RWJF-funded project, Chin explained that he and his colleagues are working with three major stakeholders—state Medicaid agencies, Medicaid managed care organizations, and frontline health care organizations—to align their efforts to use payment and care transformation to advance health equity.

Regarding the fifth lesson—to reduce disparities by framing equity as a moral and social justice issue—Chin referred to Martin Luther King, Jr.'s

1966 observation that "of all the forms of inequality, injustice in health is the most shocking and the most inhuman." "If you are trying to have other forms of human attainment, whether it's well-being, employment, education—unless you have your health, you will not be able to get there," emphasized Chin.

Chin concluded his presentation by stating that leadership matters (Chin, 2014). "It is our professional responsibility as clinicians, administrators, and policy makers to improve the way we deliver care to diverse patients," he said. "We can do better."

Disparities in Serious Illness Care for African Americans

Kimberly Johnson, associate professor of medicine and senior fellow in the Center for the Study of Aging and Human Development at the Duke University School of Medicine, began her presentation with the story of her maternal grandmother, Bertha Stokes, who was diagnosed with cervical cancer in the 1950s. Living in a small town in rural Mississippi, Stokes received care at the local hospital and then from a large public hospital in New Orleans. After several months in New Orleans, she was told there was nothing else that could be done for her, so she returned home, where she was largely cared for by her children, including Johnson's aunt. Johnson's aunt told Johnson that Stokes experienced a substantial symptom burden in the last months of her life and received little information about what to do or expect.

When Johnson's aunt recounted this story, she asked Johnson two questions. First, with all the medicines we have today, do you think she would have lived longer? Second, even if she could not be cured, do you think she would have lived better? Johnson's immediate answer was that yes, she might have lived longer, though the 5-year survival rate for cervical and uterine cancer for African American women remains lower than that for White women (see Figure 2). Johnson said the answer to the second question is uncertain because numerous studies have shown that across settings, diagnoses, and age groups, African Americans are less likely than Whites to have pain adequately assessed and treated (Meghani et al., 2012).

In addition, said Johnson, research shows that there are substantial differences in how effectively physicians communicate with patients depending on the patient's race, with African Americans receiving less information and less support than White patients, particularly in race discordant patient–physician encounters (Cooper et al., 2003; Gordon et al., 2006;

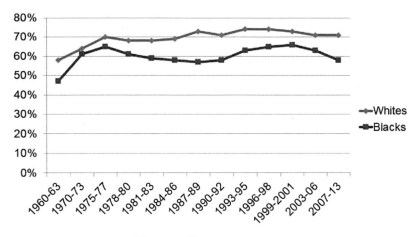

FIGURE 2 5-year survival for cervical/uterine cancer.
SOURCES: As presented by Kimberly Johnson, April 4, 2019; NCI, 2015.

Periyakoil et al., 2015; Welch et al., 2005). According to Johnson, "a Black patient and a White provider [is] the norm in our country since about only 5 percent of physicians are African American." Family members of seriously ill African American patients who die are more likely to report absent or problematic communication, explained Johnson. African Americans are also less likely to participate either formally or informally in advance care planning (ACP) (Sanders et al., 2016), which means they are less likely to talk about their preferences with providers, and even when they want to, are less likely to complete formal documentation of those preferences (Loggers et al., 2009; Mack et al., 2010). Moreover, African Americans are also less likely than Whites to enroll in hospice at the end of life (see Figure 3), an effect magnified by the fact that African Americans are more likely to suffer from cancer and heart disease, two of the more common conditions among hospice patients (Johnson, 2013).

With regard to palliative care, which did not exist in the 1950s, Johnson said that while more than 60 percent of hospitals with at least 15 beds currently have a palliative care team, the distribution of those programs is uneven across the United States. In Mississippi, for example, only 13 of 45 hospitals, and only 4 of 16 public hospitals, have a palliative care program (CAPC, 2015). This difference is important because the availability and use of palliative care has been shown to reduce disparities in hospice referral, symptom burden, discussion of treatment preferences,

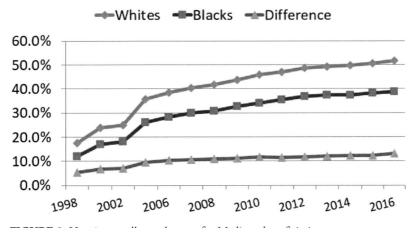

FIGURE 3 Hospice enrollment by race for Medicare beneficiaries.
SOURCES: As presented by Kimberly Johnson, April 4, 2019; MedPAC, 2004, 2011, 2012, 2013, 2014, 2015, 2016, 2017, 2018.

completion of advance directives, and use of pain medication (Sharma et al., 2015; Smith et al., 2015). "Palliative care consultation is one potential intervention to improve disparities," said Johnson (Rhodes et al., 2007).

Johnson pointed out that ACP discussions may also reduce disparities by improving communication, increasing documentation of preferences, and increasing patient and family satisfaction with the quality of communication and care (IOM, 2015). Johnson explained that she is embarking on a study, funded by the Patient-Centered Outcomes Research Institute (PCORI), to gain clarity on the extent to which ACP can reduce disparities.[9] She also noted that hospice use has been shown to reduce some disparities in terms of satisfaction with care, communication, and emotional and spiritual support received (Rhodes et al., 2007).

Johnson explained that a number of barriers still need to be addressed to make access to palliative care, hospice, and ACP more equitable, including a range of patient factors, such as knowledge about these offerings, cultural and personal preferences, spiritual beliefs, and lack of trust in the health care system. Johnson noted that other barriers include provider-related barriers, including poor communication and both explicit and implicit bias, and organizational and system barriers, such as payment

---

[9] For more information, see https://medicine.duke.edu/medicinenews/kimberly-johnson-get-58-million-pcori-contract (accessed May 28, 2019).

structures, lack of insurance, income differences, and geography (Goepp et al., 2008; Hoffman et al., 2016; Johnson, 2013).

Johnson pointed out that despite these barriers, there are opportunities to improve the care experience and reduce disparities in serious illness care through community education, outreach, and partnership with the people and institutions in the community with whom patients have their daily interactions outside of the health care system. Increased diversity of health care providers and improved cultural competency training can improve trust, interpersonal care, and access, said Johnson, who added that increased diversity among health care teams may improve health outcomes for racial and ethnic minorities (HHS Administration Bureau of Health Professions, 2016). She also noted that including nontraditional workers, such as community health workers, in the health care team can help address the barriers to equitable care (CDC NCCDPHP, 2016).

Finally, Johnson stressed that there is no uniform approach to expanding access and advancing health equity. She noted that one of the strengths of palliative care is that it emphasizes understanding people's preferences, beliefs, and values as a way to tailor personalized care for each patient.

Trauma-Informed Health Care: A Powerful Tool to Reduce Disparities in Health

"Trauma-informed care[10] is a powerful tool to address some of the most daunting challenges in medicine," said Edward Machtinger, professor of medicine and director of the Center to Advance Trauma-informed Health Care and Women's HIV Program at the University of California, San Francisco (UCSF). "It can bring healing to people with serious illnesses, it can increase satisfaction and joy for providers of care, and ultimately, it can be a pathway for us to more effectively address the disparities in health outcomes in our country," explained Machtinger.

With that introduction to his presentation, Machtinger said his awakening to the impact of trauma on health and behavior came when one of his most beloved patients, a 49-year-old African American woman with HIV named Rose, was murdered by her abusive husband. As is the case when-

---

[10] Trauma-informed health care is based on the tenet that childhood and adult trauma underline and perpetuate many serious illnesses. For more information, see https://www.capc.org/blog/palliative-pulse-the-palliative-pulse-october-2018-an-interview-with-dr-edward-machtinger-lessons-of-trauma-informed-care (accessed August 20, 2019).

ever a clinic patient died, he and the rest of the clinic's staff came together for a case conference to mourn Rose and to try to learn some lessons from the circumstances surrounding her death. This time, however, Machtinger also invited representatives from all of the agencies with which Rose had contact and all of the people who knew and loved her. What emerged from the discussions about Rose (and nine other recent patient deaths) was the realization that that the common thread across the 10 different stories was a lifelong history of trauma that led to HIV infection and eventually death. "We realized that while the biomedical focus of HIV care, like so much care for serious illnesses, is incredibly important, it is also profoundly insufficient," said Machtinger. "We realized then that we needed to transform our clinic to one that addresses trauma."

When reviewing the research on trauma and engaging in advocacy work to support this transformation, Machtinger explained that he and his colleagues realized the following:

- Most illnesses and behaviors that contribute to health disparities are correlated strongly with individual-, family-, and community-level trauma.
- Trauma continues to be an obstacle to successful treatment of many common illnesses.
- Clinics and environments of care often mirror the trauma experienced by patients and can themselves be traumatizing.

Trauma-informed care integrates these realizations into the standard of care to better address individuals' needs. To address his first realization, Machtinger explained that trauma is an event, a series of events, or set of circumstances that an individual experiences as physically or emotionally harmful or threatening and that has lasting adverse effects. These can include physical, emotional, and/or sexual abuse; neglect; loss; interpersonal or community violence; and structural violence associated with racism, sexism, homophobia, transphobia, and xenophobia (SAMHSA, 2014). He noted that the impact of trauma on adult health and well-being is well documented, citing the results of the Relationship of Childhood Abuse and Household Dysfunction to Many of the Leading Causes of Death in Adults: The Adverse Childhood Experiences (ACEs)[11] study as one example illus-

---

[11] ACEs include exposure to psychological, physical, or sexual abuse and household dysfunction, including substance abuse, mental illness, and a family member imprisoned.

trating the harms resulting from trauma (Felitti et al., 1998). Research has found that ACEs are strong predictors of the major causes of adult morbidity, mortality, and disability in the United States. For example, individuals reporting 4 or more ACEs had 1.6 times the rate of severe obesity, nearly twice the rate of heart and liver disease, twice the rate of chronic obstructive pulmonary disease and stroke, more than 3 times the rate of depression, and 10 times the rate of intravenous drug use compared to individuals reporting no ACEs (CDC, 2019a; Felitti et al., 1998).

Machtinger also referenced a study of residents in urban Philadelphia that examined the effect on health of five adverse community environments—experiencing racism, experiencing bullying, witnessing violence, being in foster care, or living in an unsafe neighborhood (Cronholm et al., 2015; Wade et al., 2016). The study found that individuals who experienced three or more of these community-level ACEs as children were more than twice as likely to smoke cigarettes as an adult or to be depressed, more than three times as likely to have a substance abuse disorder, and more than four times as likely to have a sexually transmitted disease compared to those who have not. Additionally, community-level ACEs are separate and additive from individual- and family-level traumas.

For Machtinger, these statistics shed critical light on those affected by the HIV epidemic and why his clinic's patients were dying. Specifically, he pointed out the following:

- 69 percent of people newly diagnosed with HIV are African American or Latinx[12] (CDC, 2019c).
- 30 percent of African American men who had sex with men were diagnosed with HIV (Rosenberg et al., 2014).
- 50 percent of gay and bisexual African American men are expected to be diagnosed with HIV in their lifetimes (CDC, 2019c).
- Almost one in two (44 percent) of transgender African American women are estimated to be living with HIV (CDC, 2019d).

Given that there are few meaningful biological predispositions to HIV infection, these disparities result from the lived experiences and high rates of individual-, family-, and community-level trauma experienced by African

---

[12] "Latinx" refers to a person of Latin American heritage and is used as a gender-neutral alternative to *Latino* or *Latina*. For more information, see https://www.merriam-webster.com/dictionary/Latinx (accessed July 18, 2019).

American, Latinx, and gay individuals in America, posited Machtinger. "In other words, HIV is a symptom of the much larger and more insidious reality of trauma," he said, "and the same is true for the other conditions underlying health disparities in this country." There are other examples of such disparities:

- African American women have three to four times the rate of pregnancy-related mortality (CDC, 2019e) and double the infant mortality rate compared to White women (HHS Office of Minority Health, 2017).
- Latinx children have the highest rates of childhood obesity (RWJF, 2019).
- American Indians and Alaska Natives have the highest prevalence of cigarette smoking (24 percent) compared to all other racial or ethnic groups in the United States; these groups have almost twice the rates of smoking compared to White Americans (15.2 percent) (CDC, 2019b). Native Americans have twice the rates of smoking and diabetes compared to White Americans (McLaughlin, 2010) and among the highest rates of suicide (CDC, 2018).

Trauma makes people more vulnerable to certain conditions, and it will also continue to act as an obstacle to effective treatments of those same conditions, according to Machtinger. This second realization, said Machtinger, underscores why so many medical conditions are stubbornly refractory to supposedly effective therapies. In his view, the difficulties practitioners have helping people lose weight or stop smoking, even in the face of serious health conditions, such as diabetes and lung disease, can be explained in part by the high rates of co-occurring trauma and posttraumatic stress disorder that go unrecognized and unaddressed in care plans.

Regarding the third realization—that clinics and environments of care often mirror the trauma experienced by patients—Machtinger explained that patients with a history of being abused by an intimate partner or who have had experiences in the foster care or criminal justice systems often feel unwelcome or unsafe in clinic environments. This may be because staff feel overwhelmed or unsupported and, as a result, can be dismissive, reactive, and distant from their patients. "In this way, our clinics can be trauma-inducing for patients, pushing them away from the care they need desperately," Machtinger explained.

Machtinger suggested that one plausible reason why trauma goes unaddressed in medical care is that health care professionals are trained to solve medical problems, but the sources and effects of trauma are often difficult to fix. According to Machtinger, the instinct for providers is to consider trauma as something outside of their realm of care and responsibility, meaning that this fundamental driver of disparities remains invisible.

In developing a trauma-informed clinic for HIV patients, Machtinger and his partners discovered that this model is applicable to an array of other serious illnesses. One translatable factor is the power of partnerships to break down barriers between the clinic and community organizations. These partnerships, he explained, reduce isolation for providers and offer powerful avenues of healing for patients.

Machtinger described his clinic's first partnership with Naina Khanna, executive director of the Positive Women's Network, USA,[13] which is the largest body of individuals advocating for and run by women living with HIV, according to Machtinger. Together, Machtinger and Khanna convened a national working group of 27 representatives from the military, the National Institutes of Health (NIH) and other government agencies, academia, community organizations, and individuals with lived traumatic experiences (Machtinger et al., 2015a).

The model that emerged from that convening and follow-up meetings, said Machtinger, is based on existing evidence-based interventions, expert consensus, and input from patients (Machtinger et al., 2019). It encompasses five domains (see Figure 4), with evidence-based interventions available for each domain. The challenge now, he explained, is to determine how to best package these interventions into something that can be adopted by frontline clinics and is most acceptable to providers, most efficacious, and most cost effective. Currently, Machtinger and his colleagues are collaborating with other programs across the nation on a prospective, mixed-method evaluation of the model.[14] He noted that the model builds on decades of work developing effective health system responses to intimate partner violence and that the Office of Behavioral Health Equity at the Substance

---

[13] For more information, see https://www.pwn-usa.org (accessed May 24, 2019).

[14] For more information and toolkits for this model, see https://store.samhsa.gov/product/SAMHSA-s-Concept-of-Trauma-and-Guidance-for-a-Trauma-Informed-Approach/SMA14-4884.html (accessed May 2, 2019), https://www.thenationalcouncil.org/areas-of-expertise/trauma-informed-behavioral-healthcare (accessed May 2, 2019), and http://traumatransformed.org (accessed May 2, 2019).

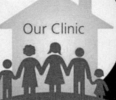

FIGURE 4 An evidence-based model for trauma-informed health care.
NOTE: IPV = interpersonal violence.
SOURCES: As presented by Edward Machtinger, April 4, 2019; Machtinger et al., 2019.

Abuse and Mental Health Services Administration has taken the federal lead on integrating trauma-informed practices into care across many fields of medicine.

Another important partnership that Machtinger's HIV clinic formed was with Rhodessa Jones, co-founder and co-artistic director of the Medea Cultural Odyssey and the Medea Project: Theater for Incarcerated Women.[15] Jones led an expressive therapy intervention with the clinic's

---

[15] For more information, see https://themedeaproject.weebly.com (accessed May 24, 2019).

patients using theater and writing. "By watching and studying her method, I learned for the first time that people can heal from even the deepest wounds of trauma, if offered the appropriate types of therapies," said Machtinger. A subsequent study of Jones's approach allowed him to better understand the ingredients for such a change that he and his colleagues are now applying to other interventions they are developing (Machtinger et al., 2015b). He noted this as an example of how a partnership within a community organization can build on the strengths of an individual's community, extend the reach of a clinic, and offer treatments and healing that differ from, and are often far deeper than, what is available in standard clinics.

Machtinger noted that another approach to addressing disparities in health is to engage and integrate peers into health care. "Peers offer opportunities for patients to support each other's healing in ways medical providers cannot and help guide the medical system's response to their own needs," said Machtinger. Integrating peers into care, he said, introduced a different way of thinking about patients and led to viewing them more as partners in their care. His clinic began engaging peers through focus groups and has moved incrementally toward a more integrated approach by including peers in bimonthly stakeholder meetings that help guide the interventions the clinic is implementing. The UCSF clinic now has a peer-led support group and peer-led intervention for co-occurring substance use and trauma and a peer-led leadership council that allows for posttraumatic growth.

An important aspect of this trauma-informed care model, Machtinger stressed, is that it is aspirational and can be implemented incrementally. "We have seen that even small steps can be felt powerfully as clinics move from being trauma-inducing to trauma-informed to trauma-reducing for patients, staff, and providers," said Machtinger. "It is hard to convey how different our clinic feels now that we have incrementally adopted each element of a trauma approach to care." He recounted how he recently saw three patients who openly discussed their struggles with cocaine addiction, and he was able to work with them to discuss ways to reduce their use of the drug. The lesson Machtinger took from these encounters was that these individuals felt safe enough in the clinic environment to reveal themselves and to ask for help. "The victory here is that it allows us as a health care clinic to more effectively address the smoking, medication non-adherence, substance use, and other trauma-related conditions that contribute to most of the disparities and health outcomes but have long been considered outside the realm of our expertise and responsibility," he added.

Concluding his remarks, Machtinger said he believes that adopting a trauma-informed approach to health care is the best way for clinicians to meaningfully address the social issues that underlie most health disparities. Trauma-informed health care, in his experience, provides a pathway to change the culture of health care to one of health equity and the nature of communication and relationships to one where patients feel safe, cared for, and respected. "If we are going to begin to dismantle health disparities in our country, we are going to need to broaden our perspective of care from one that just focuses on treating symptoms and diseases to one that includes healing," he said. As a bonus, he added, trauma-informed care can help providers heal themselves, connect better with their patients, and find joy in the process of helping people heal. In his view, such experiences are necessary for both patients and providers if the nation is ever going to make substantial progress toward reducing health disparities.

Discussion

Sarah Downer from Harvard Law School began the discussion with the panelists by asking what they thought needs to happen to change provider culture, which she called "one of the toughest nuts to crack." Chin replied that, in his experience, interactional and experiential trainings on cultural competency and health disparities have the best chance of getting health care professionals to commit to achieving health equity. For example, the course on disparities required of all first-year medical students at The University of Chicago has fewer lectures and more small group discussions and more direct contact with various diverse patient populations and communities.

The other aspect of changing provider culture, said Chin, is having a health care system that supports providers and patients. Machtinger agreed with the importance of supporting providers who are working to address the fundamental drivers of health disparities and providing them with resources and access to knowledge. At the same time, he added, health systems need to hold themselves and their providers accountable for reducing disparities. In care of patients with HIV/AIDS, for example, clinicians are held accountable for patients' viral load, but, Machtinger asserted, they should also be accountable for patients' quality of life and for factors such as depression, substance use, and other patient-centered metrics that are causing harm and sometimes leading to deaths.

Chin observed that screening for health-related social needs is increasingly popular in health care. In California, for example, there is excitement about the idea of screening for ACEs. The questions then become what to do with the resulting information, how to make sure that neither providers nor patients become overwhelmed by it, and how to use it appropriately. Machtinger posited there might not be a need for trauma screening in many patient populations because it is easy to predict that individuals seen in clinics that treat substance use disorders, mental illness, obesity, and HIV, for example, are likely to have a high burden of trauma. For the clinics that see a general population of patients, however, the added value from trauma screening is that it can help both providers and patients realize that trauma may be a key factor contributing to illnesses.

Chin commented that partnerships can expose clinicians to expertise in areas that are not traditionally part of health care. For example, health care systems should not tackle housing issues alone but should work with experts to address housing insecurity in the social services sector. What is important, he proposed, is for health care to know what role it can best play and then effectively partner with experts in those external areas that contribute to disparities and inequities.

Maguire asked the panelists to talk about the relationships they see between the social determinants of health and trauma-informed care. One difference between the two, said Hempstead, is money. Health care systems have the resources, but need to watch their bottom lines, according to Hempstead. Machtinger commented that trauma-informed care can be a helpful framework for connecting the many parallel movements in health care that seek to reduce disparities. Chin suggested that the roundtable could bring together these two fields and act as a conduit for knowledge transfer between them.

Christian Sinclair from the University of Kansas Health System and the American Academy of Hospice and Palliative Medicine remarked that as a palliative care physician, he has no power to address the social determinants of health because he sees patients when it is too late to do anything about these determinants. He noted that while he can help individuals by advocating for them with their oncologists or health systems, he was unclear what role palliative care and hospice can play to advocate for and help larger populations before they come to palliative care. Johnson replied that if the goal is to provide equitable care for people with serious illness, reaching that goal has to start with talking about equitable care further upstream. When she and her colleagues surveyed hospices about the issue, they found that hospices are thinking about it and see an opening to participate in efforts that are further upstream, such as blood pressure screenings or other kinds of chronic disease management programs in the community.

Chin remarked that health care professionals can advocate along different dimensions, starting with their own organizations and then perhaps becoming involved with national organizations. He also suggested speaking to community groups, writing commentaries for the local newspaper, and talking to elected officials.

An online workshop participant asked if there was a role for physician assistants (PAs) in addressing disparities and inequities in care. Hempstead replied that it is important for PAs to be involved with patients from the start of care so that they can form a trusted relationship with their patients. Johnson noted that the roles PAs can take varies across the nation but that she thinks of them as a part of the multidisciplinary care team, just as she does for nurse practitioners (NPs) and social workers. Chin added that there is a great untapped potential for greater involvement of PAs and NPs in serious illness care.

Denise Hess from the Supportive Care Coalition commented that, while she has great admiration for the ACEs study that Machtinger discussed, she has noticed that patients can feel stigmatized by the results of that study. That has led her to be curious about the study's outliers—individuals who had high ACE scores but defy all expectations, likely due to resilience. Hess then asked Machtinger how he incorporates resilience and growth into his work. In response to the potential stigmatization of patients, Machtinger noted that the ACE screening is not used "dispassionately," but rather serves to "awaken that provider, that clinic, and that patient, to the prevalence, the high rates of childhood traumas, and the role that that trauma is likely playing in the interaction with the health system [and] that provider, in terms of responses to therapies." He added that he has observed that when patients can understand that their behavior is a result of what happened to them rather than what is wrong with them, they blame themselves less and can start looking for solutions. He called trauma-informed care a strength-based approach because it allows patients to focus on the strengths that have sustained them despite experiences of trauma instead of their perceived failings. He added that he and his colleagues measure resilience and are trying to understand how such measures can be helpful for providers and patients moving forward. Finally, Machtinger noted that there is an emerging field of research on the physiological effects of toxic stress responses.

IMPROVING ACCESS TO CARE AND ACHIEVING
HEALTH EQUITY FOR PEOPLE WITH SERIOUS ILLNESS:
ORGANIZATIONAL AND COMMUNITY PERSPECTIVES

Nadine Barrett from the Duke University School of Medicine introduced the second session of the workshop and expressed her excitement about the continued learning opportunities she anticipated from the diverse perspectives that would be heard. Barrett pointed out that this session would focus on the organizational and community levels of the social ecological model and would address some of the opportunities and challenges in navigating the integration of serious illness care with social service and faith-based organizations.

Whole Kids Outreach: Helping to Meet the Needs
of Children with Complex Medical Problems

Sister Anne Francioni, executive director of Whole Kids Outreach,[16] led off the session by describing how her faith-based organization has been helping families with young children in rural southeast Missouri for 20 years by providing services through home visit outreach and nursing programs. Whole Kids Outreach also offers services through its physical site in Ellington, Missouri. Francioni explained that the challenge her organization faces is delivering care in a region that is socially and geographically isolated and marked by widespread poverty (U.S. Census Bureau, 2017). Children in this seven-county region in the Missouri Ozarks live in poverty and experience a high level of child abuse, neglect, and poor health as infants, according to Francioni (Missourians to End Poverty, 2018).

Francioni explained that access to pediatric specialty care is extremely limited, with the nearest facility located almost 130 miles away. Many families in the region do not have a car or the money to buy gas for a 260-mile round-trip visit to the nearest pediatrics specialty clinic, noted Francioni. Whole Kids Outreach's approach is to take evidence-based programs to the home early in a child's life. This allows the organization's NPs to both educate parents and identify some of the problems these children will face in their homes as they grow up.

---

[16] For more information, see https://wholekidsoutreach.org/#/home (accessed May 21, 2019).

Whole Kids Outreach uses Healthy Families America,[17] a trauma-informed parent education program, to teach parents how to best support their children's intellectual development, such as when to call a doctor and how to promote positive behavior without resorting to physical punishment. The basic idea, she said, is to find each family's strengths and build on those to reveal individuals' own resilience. Her organization also uses the Maternal–Child Nursing and Parents as Teachers programs,[18] two other evidence-based home visiting models. These programs aim to teach parents to teach their children by modeling desired behaviors, such as valuing education. "We are building up the person who hopefully is going to be the shaper of the culture in that family system," said Francioni. In addition to working with parents on health literacy, Whole Kids Outreach also works on building employment skills in parents to help address financial stress—an important contributor to the pressures that affect these families.

Francioni told several stories of children that Whole Kids Outreach has helped, including Marshawn, a baby born prematurely to a mother with a substance use disorder. Adopted by his foster parents, Marshawn grew into a strong young man who played basketball for his college. Eventually, Marshawn adopted a child who had been born into similar circumstances as he had been many years earlier. "You see the transgenerational problems that we can see with poverty and trauma, and you can see the transgenerational solution," said Francioni.

Francioni said that the goal of Whole Kids Outreach is to increase the health literacy and networking skills of the parents so that they can tap into the network of providers and local organizations the program has built. The network was developed in an effort to increase the odds that these parents, many of whose families have lived in poverty and neglect for generations, can change the future course of the children they raise. Francioni noted that the communities in which these parents and their children live can be remarkably supportive of families in need, so an important role played by Whole Kids Outreach is to ensure that these families are connected with their communities. To that end, the program sponsors community gatherings to help reduce social isolation, bring families together, and provide fun activities that many of these families would not otherwise be able to afford. It also has a community center in Arrington, Missouri, that offers

---

[17] For more information, see https://www.healthyfamiliesamerica.org (accessed July 2, 2019).

[18] For more information, see https://parentsasteachers.org (accessed May 22, 2019).

a horseback riding program, summer camp, children's weekend programs, youth volunteer opportunities, water safety lessons, Mom's Day Out program, and parent cafés.

Francioni also pointed out that she and her colleagues have formed collaborations with several universities outside of the area. These connections are serving as a two-way street that keep her team informed of the latest approaches for dealing with the problems these families face while facilitating the universities' efforts to engage in research with communities that are normally not accessible to them.

Familias en Acción

Adán Merecias, a community health worker with Familias en Acción[19] in Portland, Oregon, explained that the focus of the organization is to engage its community to facilitate a sharing of knowledge between community members. When Familias en Acción first opened in 1998, its mission was to provide services to Latinas dealing with domestic abuse. Its mission has since expanded, Merecias stated, to include community health workers who engage with families confronting chronic disease.

Merecias explained that community health workers, or *promotoras*, are common in Mexico and are trained to provide health education services to the communities in which they live and to engage with the community to produce better health outcomes. Similarly, Merecias sees his role as a health educator as essential to preventing disease in his community, and therefore developed Familias en Acción's community health education program. That program offers classes on diabetes, gardening, walking, and how to prepare for health care appointments. One course offering is called *Empoderamiento*[20] ("empowerment") and provides an introduction to palliative care and advance care directives. This course aids Familias en Acción's clients with serious illness by helping families to understand what questions to ask of their providers before reaching the stage where they would need palliative care services. The course also helps them identify resources that they may need access to in the community.

Merecias also worked with Kaiser Permanente to better serve Latinxs with chronic disease in his community and facilitate access to services, such

---

[19] For more information, see https://www.familiasenaccion.org (accessed May 17, 2019).

[20] For more information, see https://www.familiasenaccion.org/wp-content/uploads/2019/05/FAM_HealthClasses-2-2.pdf (accessed July 3, 2019).

as health coaches and mail-order pharmacy services. Kaiser also provided Merecias with specific training on how to engage with his clients around ACP and Kaiser's Life Care Planning program,[21] which deals with some of the social determinants of health, such as food or housing insecurity or procuring transportation to health care appointments. This latter form of planning was possible, he explained, because he went into his clients' homes and was able to learn about the home environment in a way that is not possible with clinic-based care.

As an example of the work he does, he recounted the story of one of his clients who had terminal cancer but did not understand his prognosis. His client asked him at one point if the treatments he had been receiving for many months were going to cure him. Not knowing the answer himself, Merecias offered to accompany his client to his next appointment with his oncologist and help ask his doctor to explain more about his condition and prognosis. In the end, after finally understanding that he was not going to be cured, the client made the decision to talk to his immediate family about his prognosis. He also decided to return to Mexico to spend time with his extended family, whom he had not seen for many years, before his cancer progressed to the point that he was unable to travel.

This story, Merecias said, illustrates two common roles of a community health worker: serving as a cultural bridge between the clinic and the community and as an advocate in the clinical environment. He explained that he has to tell providers that he is there with the patient as an advocate and explainer, not a language interpreter. "I am there to make sure that my client understands what is happening. I am there to make sure that they understand the diagnosis and that they have questions that they need to ask," said Merecias. "All those things need to be addressed so that they can have a better health outcome."

Merecias also told the story of Maria, a longtime volunteer with the organization. Maria worked with the Oregon food bank to modify its gardening program to make it more appropriate for her Latinx community. "Maria is a prime example of what happens when you bring somebody into an agency who is willing to learn, who has a lot of skills, but who might be willing to develop additional skills," said Merecias. "She was [not only] able … to be trained to give specific classes but … also trained in other classes

---

[21] For more information, see https://healthy.kaiserpermanente.org/health-wellness/life-care-plan (accessed July 3, 2019).

that she was able to modify so they would have a better fit for our specific community."

Chinese American Coalition for Compassionate Care

The founder of the Chinese American Coalition for Compassionate Care (CACCC),[22] Sandy Chen Stokes, explained that the organization aims to build a community in which Chinese Americans are able to face the end of life with dignity and respect. This is a simple goal, she said, but not easy to achieve, given the unique characteristics of the Chinese culture, language, and belief system. As an example, she noted that buildings in China and Taiwan do not have a fourth floor because the number four in Chinese culture is symbolic of death. "So please do not get upset if a [Chinese] family member or patient refuses to go onto the fourth floor or a room with the number four," she said. "There is a good reason—they do not want to die."

In Stokes's view, the Chinese American community needs language- and culture-appropriate services and educational materials so that its members can communicate effectively with health care providers. The community also needs to trust the members of the care team and feel that that team respects its culture. For example, elaborated Stokes, when a visiting nurse arrives at a house and does something as simple as asking if she should take her shoes off before entering, the odds are high that the family will welcome her more readily.

Having end-of-life discussions is a challenge in Chinese culture because death is a taboo subject, and, in fact, Stokes was warned that CACCC would quickly fail because of that. She and the organization have succeeded, however, using a coalition model that has engaged 150 partner organizations and 1,400 individual members who share resources, train bilingual volunteers, and educate health professionals about how to work in the context of Chinese culture. CACCC has a strong community base of volunteers trained to serve as interpreters for local health systems and to support patients and families at the end of life.

According to Stokes, one unique characteristic of the Chinese community in northern California is that the majority of all Chinese Americans in health care professions are doctors. Stokes emphasized that very few become social workers—one profession that is important to end-of-life care. This is where CACCC's large cadre of volunteers is helpful—many of them,

---

[22] For more information, see https://www.caccc-usa.org (accessed May 17, 2019).

including nurses and social workers, have participated in one of six 30-hour trainings on hospice and palliative care so that they can go into hospitals and patients' homes and provide culturally appropriate support.

One of CACCC's accomplishments has been to translate and develop Chinese end-of-life materials, including Physician's Orders for Life-Sustaining Treatment forms, the CACCC's decision aids, the educational series developed by the National Hospice and Palliative Care Organization (NHPCO) and Hospice Foundation of America, and the Conversation Project. CACCC volunteers have also created and translated a variety of books, DVDs, and short documentary films about the end of life. To raise awareness that CACCC materials are available, not just for her community in California but for all Chinese Americans, Stokes has engaged in newspaper and television campaigns and she and other CACCC volunteers regularly conduct community outreach at senior centers and other venues used by the Chinese community.

Another service CACCC offers is a Chinese volunteer hospital ambassador program. At El Camino Hospital in Mountain View, California, CACCC-trained Chinese-speaking ambassadors get a list of all Chinese-speaking patients in the hospital and visit them throughout the day. Hospital staff report that these ambassadors have been helpful in working with Chinese American patients. CACCC is in the process of expanding its ambassador program to other hospitals in the California.

Stokes sees CACCC as a bridge that connects health care providers with the Chinese community and connecting them with families and patients who are facing the end of life. One tool for helping families deal with the taboo of discussing death is CACCC's Heart-to-Heart® cards. Modeled after the Coda Alliance's Go Wish cards, each playing card contains a statement or conversation prompt about end-of-life wishes in both Chinese and English, encouraging patients to convey their wishes to family members. Each suit focuses on a different aspect of end-of-life issues—for example, hearts deal with spiritual concerns and diamonds with financial concerns. The cards are often used at Heart-to-Heart® Cafés at which people eat pastries, drink tea, and talk about end-of-life issues in a friendly, non-threatening environment.

In closing, Stokes said her goal now is to replicate what CACCC has done in other communities, not just across the country, and not just for Chinese-speaking communities. She would also like to establish partnerships with universities to research end-of-life issues among Chinese Americans.

Discussion

In the discussion following the presentations, Machtinger commented on Francioni's organization's method of involving parents in its work in an effort to interrupt generational cycles of trauma. Too often in the trauma field, he said, the focus is exclusively on children, but children do not exist in isolation. In fact, he said, an adult is involved in every ACE traditionally listed on the ACE questionnaire. For this reason, Whole Kids Outreach's focus on helping parents heal seems powerful to him. He asked Francioni how her program came to focus on adults and whether that focus creates challenges with funding or generating compassion in the community, given that troubled adults seem to trigger less compassion than troubled children. Francioni replied that her background in pediatrics is what led her to focus on adults because she knew the importance of teaching adults how to care for their seriously ill children once they leave the hospital. She sees her organization's mission as breaking the cycle that has created five generations of poor health and poverty in the area in which she works. She noted that one of the first things she does when she meets a new family is to administer an extensive parent survey that reveals the traumas they suffered as children. Then, she teaches them about the power they have to create a better life for their children and to heal themselves for the benefit of the entire family.

An online participant asked the panelists to speak about how they managed to convince the hospital decision makers to partner with their organizations to tackle the problem of health equity. Stokes said that health providers heard about CACCC's status in the community and wanted to learn more about the organization's work. Once health systems learned about the services CACCC provides to its Chinese-speaking community, they became eager to talk about partnerships. Merecias said his organization's best connection with the health system is through social workers rather than clinicians. He noted, too, that health systems in the northwestern United States are starting to recognize the positive effect community health workers can have with their patients. The main challenge his organization faces, he pointed out, is reimbursement for services.

Francioni remarked that there are no hospitals in her region in southeast Missouri, so she develops relationships with local pediatricians. Her biggest challenge is funding, and she recently had to drop three counties from her coverage area because she did not have the funds to pay nurses to work in these areas. While she would love to work with a large group of physicians and hospitals, her organization currently does not have the capacity to do so. Barrett commented that aligning priorities with those of the health care system could provide a means of tapping into reimbursement streams.

Workshop participant Thomas Quinn from Jewish Social Service Agency Hospice in Montgomery County, Maryland, asked Stokes and Merecias to speak more about how they train professionals to interact better with Chinese and Latinx communities. Stokes replied that she focuses on how to help providers communicate more effectively with Chinese-speaking patients and their families by helping them understand Chinese culture. CACCC also holds a forum at least once per year and invites community leaders and health care providers to discuss specific topics in a safe and collegial environment. Merecias noted that Familias en Acción offers training at its annual conference on how to better serve Latinxs and online and in-person training that can earn providers continuing medical education credits. The trainings concentrate on how to build rapport with Latinx patients. For example, something as simple as using the terms *señor* and *señora* can go a long way to building trust and a connection with patients and families.

Patricia Bomba from Excellus BlueCross BlueShield thanked the panelists for their consistent message about the value of bridging the community and the health care team. She also applauded the way Merecias worked with his client with terminal cancer to help him understand his prognosis and change the entire dynamic of what his goals were for the last part of his life. She suggested that the panelists examine whether their programs were having any effect on reducing unwanted hospitalizations or emergency room visits, which might open up opportunities for reimbursement.

IMPROVING ACCESS TO CARE AND ACHIEVING HEALTH EQUITY FOR PEOPLE WITH SERIOUS ILLNESS: PATIENT/FAMILY AND CLINICIAN PERSPECTIVES

The workshop's third session began with a video provided and produced by Liz Margolies, founder and executive director of the National LGBT Cancer Center, which told the story of Jay Kallio, who was age 58 and a two-time cancer patient at the time the video was made. Kallio, a transgender man who came out as a lesbian at age 12, spoke about the abuse and bullying he lived through as an adolescent. When he finally transitioned to male at age 50, he suddenly felt that as a White man, he was in a privileged position and was treated better. "I found that when I talked, people stopped interrupting me and took my ideas seriously. People accepted my authority and leadership in situations," he said.

The one caveat, he noted, was that when he had to seek medical care for cancer, his health care providers did not consider him a "real man." The result, he said, was that he would "plummet off this cliff of respect and authority I had gained with the outside world into a pit of being a freak, mentally ill, and someone who was needing psychiatric care rather than cancer care." Not long after the video was made, Kallio died from metastatic lung cancer.

Following the video, session moderator Graves commented that she also carries a great deal of privilege with her, but unlike Kallio, she has been able to bring that privilege into her health care experiences, including when she was treated for cancer. Her privilege showed, she said, every time she was viewed as assertive rather than aggressive or angry, when she insisted that her tests be done sooner rather than later, and when she gently called out her radiologist for not reading her chart prior to giving her his clinical advice. "My privilege showed when I laid face down in that breast MRI [magnetic resonance imaging] machine and the happy images that they had placed in the sightline were of three happy, smiling, White babies, when I knew I was in a predominantly African American county," Graves added.

Communication Can Drive Health Equity in Serious Illness Care

Justin Sanders, faculty member of the Serious Illness Care Program at Ariadne Labs and an attending physician in the Psychosocial Oncology and Palliative Care Department at the Dana-Farber Cancer Institute and the Brigham and Women's Hospital, spoke about the ways in which communication can drive health equity. He began his presentation by commenting on a remark that Kallio made at the end of the video: that he felt that his body was worn out from fighting discrimination, bigotry, and poverty all of his life. Sanders noted that this statement is supported by the theory of allostatic load—the cost of chronic exposure to fluctuating or heightened neural or neuroendocrine response resulting from repeated or chronic environmental challenges that are stressful to the individual. "Ample evidence supports a relationship between race and ethnicity, gender, socioeconomic status, and even social relationships on allostatic load," said Sanders.

Kallio's experiences are unfortunately not unique, and they actually characterize the experiences of many individuals with serious illness who come from marginalized communities, explained Sanders. What stands out from the interviews he conducted with community members, patients with serious illness, and bereaved caregivers in the African American community, he recalled, are the small traumas and microaggressions to which they become accustomed and the mistrust that many members of that community bring to their clinical experiences. Fortunately, he added, because good communication relates to rapport, and rapport tends to grow with mutual exposure, patients with serious illness often express a high degree of trust in their clinicians.

Health equity, he continued, is not equality—ensuring that everybody has access to the same thing—but rather means that the resources are allocated in ways that address systematic inequalities in the outcomes of clinical care. In that context, health equity in serious illness care is more than just access to a specialist or primary palliative care physician. It must also consider the outcomes around which health equity is achieved—through care that reflects the patient's goals, values, and preferences (goal-concordant care). What enables goal-concordant care, Sanders added, is communication.

Sanders and his colleagues have developed a conceptual model and approach for measuring serious illness communication and its effect on achieving goal-concordant care (Sanders et al., 2018) (see Figure 5). He explained there is a significant amount of literature and personal experience demonstrating the failure of communication for people of color and other marginalized communities. There is evidence of deficits in every one of the communication, quality, and process indicators in this model. These deficits result in people from these communities feeling less informed, less in control, and less satisfied; believing that they have a lower quality of life; and having less trust in health care institutions (Johnson, 2013; Loggers et al., 2009; Sanders et al., 2019). This is true, Sanders said, even though nationally representative studies, such as the Health and Retirement Study and the National Health and Aging Trends Study, suggest that there are no differences by race in receiving goal-concordant end-of-life care from the perspective of bereaved caregivers.

Sanders and his colleagues have been conducting interviews with bereaved caregivers of African American and White patients, and a preliminary analysis of the data yielded results that were both unsurprising and surprising. The degree to which the quality of communication reflected the quality of care was unsurprising. What was surprising, Sanders explained, was that no matter how bad communication was, no caregivers said that

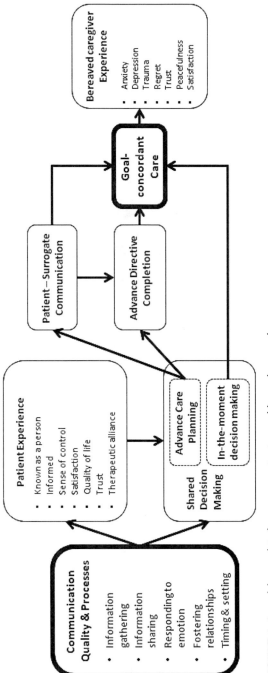

FIGURE 5 A model to explain how communication enables goal-concordant care.
SOURCES: As presented by Justin Sanders, April 4, 2019; Sanders et al., 2018.

their loved ones received care that was inconsistent with their goals. "This suggests to me that we have set a really low bar in health care for what good communication is," said Sanders. "My hope would be that people would have a goal, or an expectation at least, of experiencing communication that feels supportive and improves their illness experience."

Sanders pointed out that there is substantial evidence for individuals with serious illness that links conversations about patients' values and goals with improved quality of life, better patient and family coping, reduced anxiety and depression, enhanced goal-consistent care, more and earlier hospice care, and fewer hospitalizations at the end of life (Sanders et al., 2018; Wright et al., 2008). Sanders noted that given the multiple benefits of good communication, it is a wonder that it happens so rarely. He added that one reason is that professional training for many clinicians does not include communication skills. Clinicians can, however, be trained to communicate better, and there are a variety of programs that support clinician training in high-quality serious illness communication. "We need to incentivize clinicians to take advantage of these programs and to ensure that the innovations developed by these programs work their way into undergraduate and graduate health professional training," said Sanders.

Sanders further explained that clinicians' implicit biases, some of which are driven by an overinterpretation of what individuals from some communities do or do not want as it relates to decision making or the elements that support it, can lead to poor-quality communication. Poor communication in turn contributes to health disparities (Penner et al., 2014). Sanders compared bias to a chronic illness that may be cured in the future but is presently incurable. However, he elaborated, it can be controlled, and part of doing so involves educating clinicians about how bias can influence their interactions, their communications, and their decision making in ways that systematically affect one type of patient differently than another.

As an example of how it is possible to work with health systems to ensure that bias plays less of a role in communication and decision making, Sanders described an approach he and his colleagues at Ariadne Labs have developed. This approach, which he believes addresses discrimination and bias by attempting to ensure that every patient with serious illness has access to skilled clinician communication, involves clinical tools, clinician training and coaching, and several systems innovations to elicit and make accessible the information about patients' goals, values, and priorities. This approach includes selecting the right patients who are at risk of dying, working with them to make sure they are prepared for and expect these conversations, providing reminders to clinicians about when to have these conversations, and documenting the conversations in ways that are accessible at multiple points of care.

In thinking about ways to ensure that communication will advance health equity, Sanders noted that key issues to consider include the following:

- Are clinicians trained to initiate conversations about things that matter to patients?
- Do they feel supported to have these conversations?
- Are the conversations happening?
- Are the conversations improving patient experiences?

In Sanders's view, health systems need to spend more time focused on communication and its more proximal outcomes for patients and less time thinking about measuring goal-concordant care, around which there are many measurement complexities. "If you think about trust in the health care experience, and its correlates, such as satisfaction, I think of what we are trying to do with communication is enhance trust in systems that care for people, in part because that by itself can reduce the health systems contributions to allostatic load," explained Sanders. "We can demonstrate respect and caring through communication that enhances trust."

As a final comment, Sanders said that if health communication has systematically made people feel devalued, communication can be used to repair the relationships that have been undermined over generations. He described a Zulu greeting from South Africa: *Sawabona*, meaning "I see you." Respondents say *sikbona*, meaning, "I am here." "Communication is the cornerstone of health care that can help people feel seen. And they can say to us, with confidence, I am here," Sanders said.

Cancer Care and the LGBT Community

Margolies began her presentation by asking two questions. Is a lump a lump, or does it matter who the lump spends Valentine's Day with? Does it matter if the cancer is an ovarian tumor and the patient is a transgender man? The answer to both questions, she said, is that yes, it does matter. "We cannot separate the disease from the person it occurs in," said Margolies, adding that most intake forms do not provide people with the opportunity to disclose their sexual orientation or gender identity. At the same time, she noted, health professionals will rarely ask a patient to disclose these factors.

In a survey that asked lesbian, gay, bisexual, and transgender (LGBT) cancer patients how they declared their sexual orientation or gender identity to their health care providers, Margolies's organization found that 58 percent of respondents brought up the subject themselves, including as a way to correct a mistaken assumption made by the provider or health care worker. "That is wrong, people, and not the way it should be," she said. "It is the provider's job to create a welcoming environment and the provider's job to invite patients to bring their whole selves into treatment," she asserted. The survey also found that only 17 percent of LGBT cancer patients were asked directly about their sexual orientation or gender identity, 19 percent had the opportunity to specify these factors on a form, and 3 percent reported that someone else told their health care providers (Margolies and Scout, 2013).

This research found, too, that LGBT cancer survivors who had a partner were twice as likely to disclose their sexual orientation or gender identity. Margolies explained that many patients who said they had been out their whole lives kept their sexual orientation or gender identity a secret because the only good hospital near them was Catholic or from fear that prejudice on the part of medical care staff members might negatively affect their care (Kamen et al., 2015b; Margolies and Scout, 2013).

Margolies noted that places to record sexual orientation and gender identity are included in many electronic health records but are underused because providers need to be trained to use them and to understand that people want to be asked. One study, she said, found that 90 percent of LGBT individuals seen in the emergency department said they would answer questions about their sexual orientation and gender identity, but 77 percent of providers working in that emergency department said they would not ask that question because they believed it to be too intrusive (Haider et al., 2017).

Margolies reminded the workshop attendees that sexual orientation is unrelated to gender identity, explaining that gender identity reflects the subjective experience of one's own gender. Margolies also explained that sexual orientation refers to whom a person is attracted, but it does not provide any information about behavior. For example, a survey conducted in New York City found that 10 percent of men who identified as heterosexual and 8 percent of women who identified as lesbian had sex with a man in the prior year (IOM, 2013b; Pathela et al., 2006). She explained that knowing about behavior is important because it provides information about risks.

Cancer is generally understood as a continuum (see Figure 6), with each phase marked by different issues that are usually addressed by different providers. According to Margolies, this view is not helpful for understanding the LGBT cancer experience because of the need to disclose sexual orientation or gender identity at every phase and the fear of discrimination, barriers to care, and uneducated providers. Instead, it is more useful to understand the experience of LGBT people in terms of a circle (see Figure 7) because the issues faced by this population are not discrete but rather repeat themselves at each phase.

According to Margolies, public perception is that LGBT discrimination ended with the advent of marriage equality, but this is inaccurate. She explained that in 2016, lesbian, gay, and bisexual people were the second largest target of hate crimes, surpassed only by African Americans (Levin et al., 2018). However, she added, the LGBT community is diverse and discrimination is not distributed equally, with transgender women of color, for example, having the greatest risk of being murdered (Park and Mykhyalyshyn, 2016), while 70 percent of transgender individuals have been harassed in restrooms. This harassment can have severe health consequences: some transgender individuals have chosen not to drink water so that they do not have to use a public bathroom, leading to dehydration and kidney problems (Herman, 2013).

Margolies noted that lesbian, gay, and bisexual individuals in states without protective policies are five times more likely than those in other

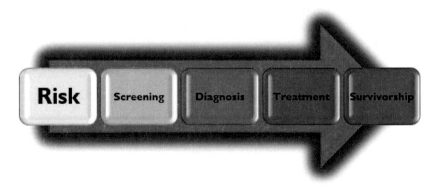

FIGURE 6 The cancer continuum, with each phase marked by different issues that are usually addressed by different providers.
SOURCES: As presented by Liz Margolies, April 4, 2019; adapted from IOM, 2013a.

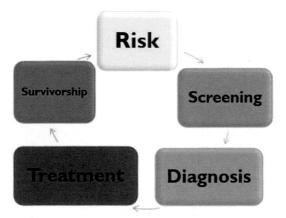

FIGURE 7 The cancer experience of LGBT individuals, reflecting that the challenges they face are not limited to one phase.
SOURCE: As presented by Liz Margolies, April 4, 2019.

states to have two or more mental disorders (Hatzenbuehler et al., 2009). She added that those who had experienced prejudice-related major life events were three times more likely to have suffered a serious physical health problem during the subsequent year, regardless of age, gender, employment, and even health history. Other increased health risks in this population are a result of increased rates of eating disorders, obesity, and tobacco use and drug use (Garcia, 2014).

Even with the passage of the Patient Protection and Affordable Care Act (ACA), which Margolies explained was beneficial to the LGBT community, LGBT individuals are still much more likely to be uninsured than their non-LGBT peers and LGBT women are twice as unlikely to have a personal health care provider (Gates, 2014). A Harris Interactive Poll found that 75 percent of lesbians delayed obtaining health care, and 16 percent of those reported that the reason for such a delay was that they were concerned about discrimination (Harris Interactive, 2005).

Regarding the lack of provider knowledge about LGBT health issues, Margolies said that medical school and nursing school education include an average of only 5 (Obedin-Maliver et al., 2011) and 2 (Lim et al., 2015) hours dedicated to LGBT health, respectively. As a result, she said, 50 percent of transgender and gender non-conforming people have had to teach their medical providers about transgender care, and nearly 20 percent of them have been refused care because they were transgender or gender non-conforming (Grant et al., 2011). In addition, more than 80 percent of first-year medical students express implicit bias against lesbian or gay individuals and nearly half expressed explicit bias (Burke et al., 2015), while heterosexual nurses held strong implicit preferences for heterosexual people over gay and lesbian people (Sabin et al., 2015).

Margolies noted that given that tumor registries do not collect information about gender identity or sexual orientation, it is hard to say whether LGBT individuals suffer from more cancer than the general population. "I can tell you that we smoke at rates that are about 40 percent higher than the general population, but I cannot tell you anything about the rates of lung cancer in LGBT people," said Margolies. What data are available, she said, show that 14 percent of lesbians and 17.6 percent of bisexual women have reported ever having had cancer compared to 11.9 percent for heterosexual women and that bisexual women have the highest rate of breast cancer at 8.4 percent (Alexander et al., 2016). Lesbians also have higher 5-year and lifetime risks for developing breast cancer (Dibble et al., 2004), while gay men are 44 times more likely than men in the general population to be diagnosed with anal cancer (Dandapani et al., 2010). Only 1.8 percent of research funded by NIH and focused on sexual and gender minorities goes toward cancer research, compared with 75 percent for HIV/AIDS research (NIH Sexual and Gender Minority Research Coordinating Committee, 2015). "If funding and research on LGBT populations and cancer continue at this pace, then we are decades away from understanding and eventually alleviating the cancer burden among LGBT populations," said Margolies.

Once diagnosed, LGBT individuals face additional challenges, including more distress, fair or poor health, and lower satisfaction with care (Boehmer et al., 2011; Kamen et al., 2015a). Gay, bisexual, and transgender men have reported more psychological distress after surviving cancer than their straight peers, and compared with the general male population, gay men with prostate cancer reported significantly worse functioning and more severe bother scores on urinary, bowel, and hormonal symptom scales; worse mental health functioning; and greater fear of cancer recurrence (Hart et al., 2014; Kamen et al., 2015a).

Margolies explained that many LGBT people are wary of the health care system and avoid engagement with it as much as possible. Given that research indicates that disclosure of sexual orientation or gender identity is related to improved safety and better health outcomes (Durso and Meyer, 2013), the finding that gay and lesbian patients—and particularly older ones—have considerable difficulty disclosing their sexual identity to cancer care providers is particularly problematic, according to Margolies (Brotman et al., 2003; Katz, 2009).

Margolies emphasized that support systems for LGBT individuals differ from those of the general population, where most people have partners or relatives to help with their care. Many LGBT individuals are alienated from their families, and rely on their "families of choice," made up of friends and ex-partners. She explained that, LGBT people are twice as likely to be caregivers than their cisgender and heterosexual counterparts and they are more likely to be caregivers for their neighbors (Deni, 2012), which was very common in the early years of the HIV/AIDS epidemic. In closing, she noted that her organization has developed reports on best practices in cancer care for LGBT individuals.[23]

A View from the Safety Net: San Francisco Health Network

Alice Huan-mei Chen, chief medical officer and deputy director of the San Francisco Health Network (SFHN) and professor of medicine at UCSF, began the final presentation by reminding the workshop of the bidirectional relationship between health and poverty. Poverty affects access to care and the environment in which one lives. That environment can increase exposure to health hazards, such as lead paint and pollution, and limit access to fresh fruits and vegetables. In addition, poorer neighborhoods are disproportionately targeted for marketing efforts by tobacco and alcohol companies, which contributes to individual behaviors that negatively affect health. At the same time, poor health is a contributor to poverty through profound effects on educational and employment opportunities, as well as medical debt. Chen pointed out that the top 1 percent of American men in terms of income live 15 years longer, on average, than men in the bottom 1 percent; in women, that difference is 10 years (Khullar and Chokshi, 2018).

This bidirectional relationship, Chen said, underscores the critical role of the safety net[24] in ensuring access to and equity in health care. For better or worse, said Chen, safety net systems are now more important than ever given that Medicaid covers one in five Americans (Kaiser Family Founda-

---

[23] For more information, see https://cancer-network.org/reports/lgbt-best-and-promising-practices-throughout-the-cancer-curriculum (accessed May 8, 2019).

[24] The IOM defines the safety net as providers that organize and deliver a significant level of health care and other needed services to uninsured, Medicaid, and other vulnerable patients. For more information, see https://www.nap.edu/catalog/9612 (accessed July 8, 2019).

tion, 2018a), one in three Californians (California Health Care Foundation, 2019), and four out of every nine individuals with disabilities (Kaiser Family Foundation, 2018a). "If you are someone with a serious illness and disability, four out of nine are covered by Medicaid," said Chen. "This is not a niche program. This is a major piece of our health care system."

As an example of the population served by the safety net, Chen shared the story of one of her patients, a 61-year-old Spanish-speaking woman with severe deforming lupus who lived with her 88-year-old mother and 23-year-old daughter in a single room. All three shared a decrepit bathroom and small kitchen with several other people who rented rooms on the same floor. Her patient was the full-time caregiver for her mother, who had not left the room for months, even to go to the bathroom. She served meals at a local school once per week, in part so that she could get a free lunch, said Chen. Chen explained that over the prior 2 years, insurance problems restricted her access to her lupus medications for weeks at a time, causing her lupus to worsen and make it much harder for her to care for her mother.

Chen thinks of her safety net patients as the "canaries in the coal mine": they have more vulnerabilities than individuals in the general population, but the issues they face are present in every system. In her health care system, for example, 30–35 percent of patients seen in the primary care safety net setting have difficulty finding a job, 35–40 percent experience food insecurity, and nearly 40 percent have difficulty paying bills (see Figure 8).[25] Approximately 80 percent are covered by Medicaid, including those also covered by Medicare (Chen, 2019).[26] While the needs of patients in safety net systems can seem overwhelming, there are good interventions that can serve as a buffer for them, said Chen.

For example, regarding providing universal access to health care, San Francisco established Healthy San Francisco[27] in 2007, a program that ensures universal access to health care for any adult resident of San Francisco with an income up to 500 percent of the federal poverty level, regardless of preexisting conditions or documentation status. Upon enrollment, beneficiaries of the program receive a primary care provider and a network of care that includes specialists, diagnostics, and pharmacy coverage. At its peak, said Chen, around 65,000 people enrolled in the program. Since the passage of the ACA, California and San Francisco have been diligent about getting

---

[25] This text has been revised since prepublication release.

[26] These data are based on the UCSF hospital system's internal electronic medical records.

[27] For more information, see https://healthysanfrancisco.org (accessed May 21, 2019).

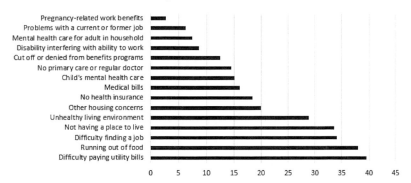

FIGURE 8 Individuals seen in safety net systems have a multiplicity of needs, based on a survey of approximately 1,000 parents of children treated in a safety net pediatric clinic.
SOURCES: As presented by Alice Huan-mei Chen, April 4, 2019; data from Laura Gottlieb based on the UCSF hospital system's internal electronic medical records.

eligible individuals to enroll in Medicaid or Covered California, the state's health insurance exchange. As a result, fewer than 14,000 people are now enrolled in Healthy San Francisco (Kauffman, 2017). While Chen's patient with lupus had gaps in her prescription coverage, Chen had the assurance that Healthy San Francisco would cover the lupus medications, if needed.

SFHN screens its patients for race, ethnicity, language preference and proficiency, sexual orientation, and gender identity, said Chen. "What we do not do, surprisingly, is systematically screen for all those social needs, partly because you are opening a can of worms with that." Instead, SFHN is implementing an enterprise electronic health record system, which includes the means to record health-related social needs. This capability will enable SFHN to collect data on health-related social needs that are more prevalent and pressing for its patients. Data are necessary but not sufficient to address disparities in care, said Chen, so SFHN has established primary care behavioral health teams to address disparities (see Figure 9).

Behavioral health clinicians do short-term counseling for issues such as stress reduction, sleep problems, depression, smoking cessation, and elder or child abuse. Behavioral health assistants, meanwhile, address health-related social needs such as housing, food, transportation, and in-home resources.

48

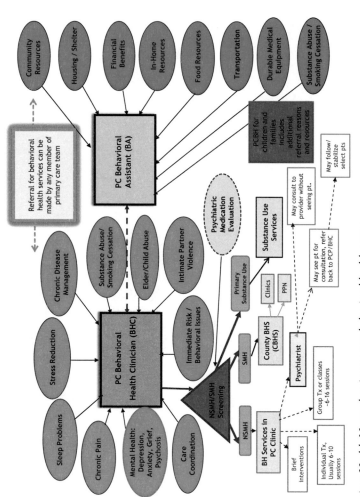

FIGURE 9 San Francisco Health Network primary care behavioral health teams.

NOTE: BHS = behavior health services; NSMH = non-specialty mental health services; PC = primary care; PCP = primary care provider; PPN = private provider network; SMH = specialty mental health services.

SOURCE: As presented by Alice Huan-mei Chen, April 4, 2019.

"While we are not there yet, our goal is to do universal screening and connection," said Chen.

Of all of the health-related social needs these patients experience, Chen considers food insecurity to be the most egregious and also one that health systems should be able to address. However, she said, health systems have only recently realized the extent to which Americans are food insecure. Across the United States, 12 percent of households are food insecure, said Chen, with that figure doubling in Latinx and African American children (Bauer, 2018; Feeding America, 2019). Chen noted that in her primary care clinics, food insecurity can reach 40 percent with many individuals living in food deserts. As an example, Chen described one of her patients, a 56-year-old man with poorly controlled diabetes. She said his vegetable intake consisted of home-fried potatoes, canned corn, and canned green beans. He had never tasted broccoli, cauliflower, or Brussels sprouts, and while he was willing to eat lettuce and tomatoes, they were not available in his neighborhood.

To serve other people in similar circumstances, many health care systems have started food pharmacies, though Chen is not convinced that the health care system is well-equipped to be a food purveyor. Still, she believes health systems have an important role to play with regard to raising the visibility of food insecurity and food deserts. SFHN has food pharmacies at its hospital and several clinics, coupled with nutrition services, cooking demonstrations, and linkages to other food resources. She noted that a study conducted in San Francisco in partnership with the nonprofit Project Open Hand has shown that giving food to food insecure HIV patients increased their antiretroviral medication adherence from 47 to 70 percent (Palar et al., 2017). Based on that result and similar findings from a study in Philadelphia (Irving, 2019), the California legislature allocated $6 million over 3 years for a trial of providing 90 days' worth of medically tailored meals to 1,000 patients who have been hospitalized with congestive heart failure or diabetes (Gorn, 2018). The outcomes of the trial will include emergency department visits, hospitalizations, and days spent in skilled nursing facilities.

Chen's final comments addressed the digital divide. She noted that although technology has incredible potential to transform how health care systems interact with their patients and to empower patients, there is also the risk of leaving people behind. As a result of limited English proficiency and health literacy, UCSF's patients may have trouble navigating a patient portal and gleaning useful information from it, she explained. To address this disparity, Chen indicated that UCSF has developed basic in-person and video-based trainings in multiple languages and enrolled proxies, or individuals who can serve as bridges between the portal and patient.

Discussion

Judy Salerno, president of The New York Academy of Medicine, commented that when she met recently with a group of medical students from New York City, they were concerned that they were not being educated about how to deal with non-medical issues that affect their patients' health, such as housing and food insecurity. As a result, they felt helpless when encountering patients with those issues and wanted information on how to advocate for their patients. She called on the workshop participants to think about how to support medical students' training so that they can help empower their future patients and confront the issues that have a significant effect on their patients' health. Philip Pizzo from Stanford University made a similar plea, noting that every National Academies panel he had served on addressed the failure of efforts to teach providers the appropriate skills to deal with these issues—indicating that it is likely a systemic failure in educational processes.

Chen responded that it is critical for future clinicians and health care professionals to be educated about these social needs. Too often, she sees patients who come to the clinic because of high blood pressure when their most pressing issue is food or housing insecurity or immigration status. She also noted that it should not be the sole responsibility of the individual provider or even the health care system to fix this problem. Rather, any solution must be team-based and include community-based partners. At the macro level, said Chen, money spent on early educational and poverty reduction interventions will provide a larger return in health than putting that money into hospitals and clinics.

Margolies, a trained social worker, added that she was happy to hear that the answer was not "call the social worker." For too long, she said, all social issues have been the responsibility of social workers and not integrated into the delivery of care. Graves remarked that efforts to educate students should incorporate social issues throughout the curriculum rather than in separate coursework.

Machtinger agreed with all of these points and asked if, from a strategy perspective, there was a way to better align various movements toward achieving the same goal, which is helping to serve all communities better.

Chen replied that while there is a great deal of misalignment among efforts to reduce disparities and inequities, she believes there is starting to be convergence around these larger structural issues. Sanders added that health systems have come to realize that improving their ability to communicate effectively with all of their patients can improve quality of care and reduce costs, while also addressing health equity. Chen commented that the recent increase in interest about health-related social needs and individual-level social determinants of health are being driven by accountable care organizations and cost savings.

Both Anne Keleman from the District of Columbia's Washington Hospital Center and Marian Grant, senior regulatory advisor at the Coalition to Transform Advanced Care (C-TAC), asked the panelists if they knew of any approaches for dealing with chronic bias in the health care system. Sanders replied that the Vital Talk program,[28] which targets clinicians, works to change practice and that his hope is that this filters down to students. Margolies said addressing bias comes down to developing better, culturally competent communication skills and changing attitudes. "You can teach people how to say the right thing, but it is really the attitude that is going to make the biggest difference," she said. As a final comment, James Tulsky, vice chair of the roundtable, wondered if serious illness care can serve as a type of pilot project to work on the issues the panel raised and incorporate solutions into the models of care being built around serious illness care.

A POLICY AGENDA TO IMPROVE ACCESS TO CARE AND ACHIEVE HEALTH EQUITY FOR PEOPLE WITH SERIOUS ILLNESS

As an introduction to the workshop's penultimate session, Sarah Downer, associate director of Whole Person Care and instructor at Harvard Law School's Center for Health Law and Policy Innovation, noted that chronic illness is the lens through which the Center focuses its efforts to use law and policy as a means of improving access to care and quality of care for underserved populations. Her work deals specifically with identifying the types of services that will make health care work better for people with complex conditions and how to use the policy level of the social ecological model to change the system to ensure that these services can meet the needs of those who have complex health conditions.

---

[28] For more information, see https://www.vitaltalk.org (accessed May 21, 2019).

Downer said the Center, with the California Food is Medicine Coalition, strongly advocated for the state to set aside money for the pilot that Chen discussed to provide medically tailored meals. The advocacy effort also emphasized team-based care that includes covering the services of community health workers and other nontraditional health care professionals. One challenge for achieving health care reform that she identified is figuring out how to fund the community-based organizations that are doing the job of improving equity in the health care system.

Addressing Disparities for Vulnerable Populations

Diane Rowland, executive vice president of the Henry J. Kaiser Family Foundation, opened her remarks by discussing possible approaches for expanding access to Medicaid. In her opinion, the strategy would include increasing access to home- and community-based services (HCBS), reducing institutional care, reducing state-to-state variability in services, facilitating integration of services, and closing the coverage gap for the 2.5 million adults who are below the poverty level yet lack access to coverage through either Medicaid or the ACA (Garfield et al., 2019).

Regarding efforts to increase eligibility for HCBS offered to Medicaid beneficiaries, Rowland applauded Congress's bipartisan work to reauthorize the spousal impoverishment provisions and permanently apply the associated rules to HCBS.[29] It is also important to maintain federal Medicaid matching funds with no preset limit and offer enhanced funds for states to cover HCBS, according to Rowland. She said that work is needed to help shore up the direct care workforce with wage increases and workforce development strategies. Too often, she said, home-based health workers themselves are impoverished because they are paid so poorly (Shierholz, 2013).

Many states, said Rowland, are looking at how to increase housing supports that can keep those with serious illness in the community, which would be helped by reauthorizing the federal Money Follows the Person demonstration[30] that offered housing-related services and staff to support people moving from nursing homes to the community. However, she added

---

[29] For more information, see https://www.congress.gov/congressional-record/2019/03/25/house-section/article/H2773-1 (accessed July 9, 2019).

[30] For more information, see https://www.macpac.gov/publication/money-follows-the-person-demonstration-program (accessed May 21, 2019).

that that would also create a need for quality measures to monitor and evaluate progress in rebalancing long-term services and supports (LTSS), how well patients are integrated into the community, and whether they improve beneficiaries' quality of life.

To illustrate the varying coverage of HCBS, Rowland noted that in 2017, 4.6 million seniors and people with disabilities used Medicaid HCBS at a cost of $82 billion. However, 86 percent of the enrollment and 93 percent of the spending went to services provided at a state level (Musumeci et al., 2019b) (see Figure 10). "Where you live determines what you get in terms of services and what waivers are available," said Rowland. The only thing available in all states, she added, is Medicaid's mandatory home health care services benefit, which leads to people in some states waiting years to receive those services (Musumeci and Watts, 2019; Musumeci et al., 2019a). In addition, the only groups eligible for that service in every state are Supplemental Security Income beneficiaries or those who come through Medicare savings programs. While most states do cover children with significant disabilities, coverage for everyone else is variable across states (Musumeci et al., 2016) (see Figure 11). Rowland noted that in her view, the home- and community-based benefit needs to be further expanded to reduce the reliance of many states on the mandatory Medicaid nursing home benefit (see Figure 12).

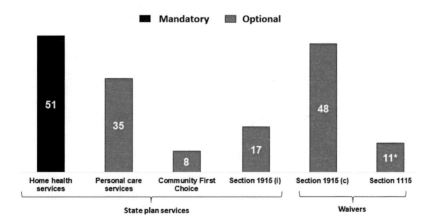
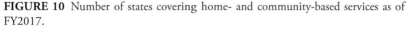

FIGURE 10 Number of states covering home- and community-based services as of FY2017.
NOTE: *Includes states within Section 1115 HCBS waivers without any accompanying Section 1915 (c) waivers.
SOURCES: As presented by Diane Rowland, April 4, 2019; Musumeci et al., 2019b.

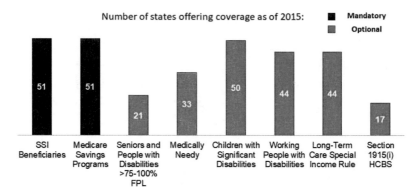

FIGURE 11 Most Medicaid eligibility pathways for seniors and people with disabilities are optional for states.

NOTES: The federal poverty level (FPL) for an individual in 2015 was $11,770; HCBS = home- and community-based services; SSI = Supplemental Security Income.

SOURCES: As presented by Diane Rowland, April 4, 2019; Musumeci et al., 2016.

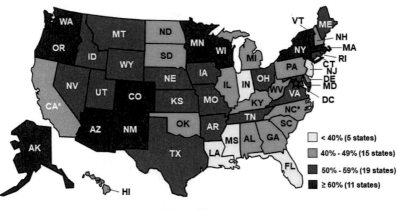

FIGURE 12 Share of total FY2016 Medicaid spending on LTSS devoted to home- and community-based health care.

NOTE: California was excluded from this figure because a high proportion of LTSS were delivered through managed care and detailed managed care information was not available for FY2016.

SOURCES: As presented by Diane Rowland, April 4, 2019; data from Eiken et al., 2018.

One issue that complicates efforts to improve services, said Rowland, is that a majority of states now deliver Medicaid LTSS through capitated managed care plans (Kaiser Family Foundation, 2019a). However, according to Rowland, state implementation of Medicaid-managed LTSS can be complex given the lack of community housing, workforce shortages, and difficulty in setting payment rates, engaging providers, selecting quality measures, and providing person-centered planning.

Rowland noted that a coverage gap exists for much of the low-income population, particularly among minorities, in the 14 states that have chosen to not participate in Medicaid expansion (Kaiser Family Foundation, 2019b). In those states, many individuals below 100 percent of the federal poverty level (FPL) are not eligible for Medicaid. For example, in Texas, the annual income limit for parents in a family of three is $3,626, despite the fact that the FPL is $21,330 (Kaiser Family Foundation, 2019c). Rowland added that this gap is also reflected in the lack of coverage for low-income childless adults, many of whom are at risk if they become seriously ill (Brooks et al., 2019). "Medicaid has some challenges to broaden, to improve, and to fill in the gaps," said Rowland.

There are opportunities to make Medicare more affordable, including capping catastrophic coverage for Part D, which the National Academies recommended (NASEM, 2018), broadening supplemental coverage through Medicaid, providing options for high-cost and high-need populations, and filling benefit gaps. The Medicare Part D benefit, she explained, has no annual limit on out-of-pocket costs, which means that even after beneficiaries reach the catastrophic cap, they still have a 5 percent copay on drugs (Kaiser Family Foundation, 2018b). In 2016, nearly 10 percent of Medicare Part D enrollees had drug spending above the catastrophic coverage threshold, and while subsidies were available for some beneficiaries, 1 million individuals were not subsidized (Cubanski et al., 2017, 2018b) (see Figure 13). Many of the drugs that cause beneficiaries to exceed the catastrophic cap, she explained, are for treating cancer (Cubanski et al., 2019).

Rowland noted that 6.1 million people, or 19 percent of the Medicare population, do not have supplemental coverage for cost sharing (Cubanski et al., 2018a). She asked whether there are ways to broaden Medicaid coverage for low-income Medicare beneficiaries, such as by raising the asset limit so that more people with low incomes but some assets could qualify. Another area that needs attention, according to Rowland, concerns people in Medicare Advantage Plans who want to switch back to traditional Medicare when they become seriously ill and would prefer

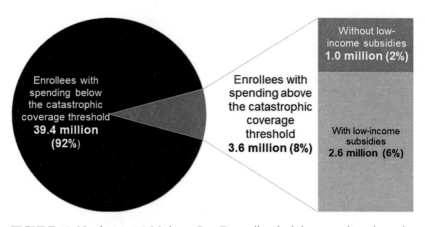

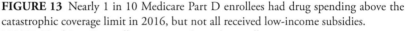

FIGURE 13 Nearly 1 in 10 Medicare Part D enrollees had drug spending above the catastrophic coverage limit in 2016, but not all received low-income subsidies.
NOTE: Total Part D enrollment in 2016 was 43.0 million.
SOURCES: As presented by Diane Rowland, April 4, 2019; information from Kaiser Family Foundation analysis of 2016 prescription drug claims data from the CMS Chronic Conditions Data Warehouse.

to receive care from an out-of-network provider. In many states, she said, they are considered to have preexisting conditions and are thus prohibited from accessing Medigap coverage. She pointed out that this locks people into their Medicare Advantage Plan, which may help them with their cost sharing but may not gain them access to the kind of specialty care that they want and need. Rowland stated that only Connecticut, Maine, Massachusetts, and New York require Medigap insurers to offer policies to all beneficiaries age 65 or older, either continuously or during the annual enrollment period, regardless of any preexisting conditions (Boccuti et al., 2018). She added that addressing Medicare's benefit gaps may assist in addressing the needs of beneficiaries with serious illness.

Rowland recounted the story of a family that had a member being treated for cancer. The family suffered economically because another family member had to quit work to care for that person. "When we look at the economic cost of serious illness, we need to broaden the lens to look at how much providing that support costs in addition to what health care programs cover and what they do not," advocated Rowland.

In closing, Rowland emphasized that she believes the people who are most in need of assistance are often those with the fewest resources and lowest incomes. Individuals from marginalized communities and who live in medically underserved areas are disproportionately in need, she pointed out.

Addressing the High Cost of Serious Illness Care

The life course today for many Americans includes an accumulation of chronic conditions, said Andrew Slavitt, founder and general partner of Town Hall Ventures and former acting commissioner of CMS, but the U.S. health care system is largely set up to meet acute needs and offer some primary care rather than addressing chronic conditions. This has led to an environment in which many people in America cannot afford to get sick. As examples, Slavitt noted that one in four Americans say it is difficult to afford their prescriptions (Kirzinger et al., 2019) and that 42 percent of individuals diagnosed with cancer will have spent all of their life savings within the next 2 years (Gilligan et al., 2018).

Slavitt also commented on the disparities in health care and how they translate into poor outcomes, using maternal mortality as an example: the United States has the highest rate of maternal mortality among high-income countries (Gunja et al., 2018). However, the data for African American women show the United States is doing as poorly as Mexico and Uzbekistan, "where significant proportions of the population live in poverty" (Roeder, 2019). "If we focus on averages, not only do we miss the problem, but we miss the opportunity to focus on solutions," said Slavitt, "and so we create a system that treats the average, which means we do a pretty horrible job of treating the people who really need it."

The reasons for this and other disparities in health outcomes include social factors being grouped together under "social determinants of health," but it also reflects biases in how the providers treat people in the health care system and how that care looks at the social determinants, argued Slavitt. In his opinion, the U.S. health care enterprise needs to reimagine its role in addressing the social determinants of health if the goal is to keep people healthy rather than treating them when they are sick. "Maybe we can play some sort of a more central role in the community that focuses on some of these other issues," said Slavitt.

According to Slavitt, when a person cannot afford to take care of a sick family member, it triggers an existential crisis. "You do not feel like an adequate parent, and you do not feel like you could capably lead a middle-class life," said Slavitt. "When someone threatens that, whether it is an insurance company's fine print, an administration, a Congress, a judge, or anybody else, that threat is an existential threat to people, and I think we have seen why health care has become not just a life-and-death issue for people but quite a big pocketbook issue." The bottom line, he added, is that health care is the underpinning to someone's ability to live a middle-class life. He added that few Americans, whether insured or not, are certain that they will be able to pay for the care they need if something horrible happens to their health (The Commonwealth Fund, 2008).

Slavitt then listed three principles that he thinks should underlie how the nation structures and pays for health care. First, if people are healthy, they can work, but they should not have to work to be able to get healthy. Second, the more we can connect dollars to patient care, the better. Disassociating money from the treatment in the health care system correlates with decreasing the importance of accountability. He argued that funding pools, such as block grants, break the connection between dollars and health care, with the result that accountability and value-based care will matter less to those making policy decisions about how to pay for health care. Lastly, he elaborated that insurers should not decide who and what gets covered. They really do not want that responsibility. "This is not a pro-government/ anti-government point," explained Slavitt. "They just want a set of rules they can follow."

Slavitt noted that studies show that more and more new jobs do not offer health care insurance today (Kaiser Family Foundation, 2017). For those that do, employees spend a significant portion of their salaries on insurance premiums, even before the money they will have to spend on the deductible and copays. He believes there needs to be a national discussion on what reasonable measures of patient responsibility should be and that there is room for disagreement.

Slavitt pointed out that there will be tough decisions to make and it will be necessary to address the special interest groups that are maintaining the status quo. "They will adjust, but we have to have the patient voice at the table, not just the special interest voice," said Slavitt.

In closing, Slavitt observed that he believes there are certain aspects of health care that should be a public good, such as insulin and ambulances, and he cautioned against putting too much stock in value-based care as the solution to the issues of cost of care. "I have always believed that payments are not going to dictate high-quality care," said Slavitt. "Culturally sensitive leadership focused on quality and commitment should do that, and payments ought to support and reward that," he concluded.

Policy Approaches to Improving Access to
Care for People with Serious Illness

In the session's final presentation, Lori Bishop, vice president of palliative and advanced care at NHPCO, discussed three approaches that her organization is taking to improve access to and equity of care for people with serious illness.

The first approach involves support for new payment and delivery models, including the alternative payment model for Medicare beneficiaries with serious illness that CMS is expected to announce. This limited-scale demonstration project is expected to include provisions that will promote interdisciplinary care, whole-person and family-centered care, and 24-hour access to care. "Those are key components of a model that has worked really well for years, and that happens to be a hospice model of care," said Bishop. Her hope is that the demonstration project will include a cross-section of the American public and not just one demographic group.

Bishop discussed the second approach, which focuses on several new pieces of legislation, including the Rural Access to Hospice Act[31] and the Palliative Care and Hospice Education and Training Act.[32] The Rural Access to Hospice Act, introduced in April 2017, would increase access to underserved Medicare beneficiaries in rural areas and at federally qualified or community health centers (NHPCO HAN, 2017). Currently, she explained, there is a disincentive for physicians in rural areas or who work at a community health center to refer patients to hospice because they are then no longer reimbursed for the care they provide for their patients. She noted this bill has bipartisan support but that it keeps getting added on to bills that lack such support (GovTrack.us, 2019).

The Palliative Care and Hospice Education and Training Act, which the House passed with bipartisan support, would address the workforce shortage that everyone acknowledges will limit specialty care, and perhaps even primary care, in the near future. She said that some estimates are for no more than a 1 percent growth rate in the palliative care and hospice workforce over the next 20 years, while the number of people eligible for palliative care is projected to grow by more than 20 percent (Kamal et al.,

---

[31] For more information, see https://www.congress.gov/bill/115th-congress/senate-bill/980 (accessed May 21, 2019).

[32] For more information, see https://www.congress.gov/bill/115th-congress/house-bill/1676 (accessed May 21, 2019).

2017). Bishop described this bill as comprehensive in its support for education and its funding for research.

The third approach that Bishop discussed involves looking at independent and innovative ways to eliminate the barriers to the hospice model of care so that people with serious illness can have timely access to person-centered, interdisciplinary care. One way to do that might be through structural reform of the Medicare hospice benefit, which is something NHPCO is studying. For example, the hospice benefit requires that a patient has less than 6 months to live, but after 40 years of hospice, nobody has yet developed a way to prognosticate when that 6-month period starts, according to Bishop. She noted the Medicare Care Choices[33] demonstration model for concurrent care is something NHPCO would like to see approved and allowed for all patients, though the question of how to pay for this benefit has yet to be solved. One thought is to provide palliative care further upstream from hospice in a continuum of care model. "So, you might get the intensive hospice care for a shorter period of time overall, but you get it at the point when you need it," she explained.

NHPCO is also working to define what community-based palliative care is to make it easier for policy makers to decide how to pay for it. She noted that California has implemented a new law, which has language on basic expectations of care for the state's Medicaid population and could serve as a template for congressional action.

In closing, Bishop noted that NHPCO collaborated with the We Honor Veterans program[34] on a trauma-informed care program that offers veterans nearing the end of life the opportunity to talk about experiences they have never shared before. Bishop pointed out that NHPCO is using the learnings from this program to develop its Equity at the End of Life program, which aims to increase diversity and inclusion for marginalized populations within hospice.

Discussion

The discussion session following the speakers' presentations began with Cheryl Matheis of C-TAC asking each panelist to suggest one thing the field could focus on to improve access and advance equity. Rowland pro-

---

[33] For more information, see https://innovation.cms.gov/initiatives/medicare-care-choices (accessed May 17, 2019).

[34] For more information, see https://www.wehonorveterans.org (accessed May 17, 2019).

posed fixing the Medicare Part D cap to protect the millions of people who exceed it each year and give some sense of security to those who take costly specialty drugs. Slavitt offered that there may be a near-term opportunity to take bipartisan action on prescription drug costs, which would significantly benefit a large number of people. Bishop recommended restructuring the hospice benefit for the seriously ill so that more people could get access to holistic care and then receive timely and appropriate access to the full benefit of hospice when they need it. She shared her concern that hospice care is being addressed from the perspective of a business model rather than a care model.

Bomba had two questions about the Rural Access to Hospice Act. The first was whether NPs who operate independently, in the states where that is allowed, will be able to authorize hospice, and the second was whether the bill includes funds that would help rural hospice programs provide comprehensive care. Bishop replied that the problem with not allowing NPs to authorize hospice affects all geographical areas, not just rural areas, and that changing regulations to permit NPs and PAs to do so is not included in the rural health care bill. She said that addressing this issue is going to be a long battle that will require a concerted effort on the part of the community to convince policy makers of the need to make that change and pass the Removing Barriers to Person- and Family-Centered Care Act of 2019.[35]

Chin commented that he would have liked if the speakers had offered solutions that directly attacked the problem of health equity and disparities for diverse populations beyond what appears to be a "rising tide lifts all boats" approach. Rowland responded that work on disparities that her organization has done shows that the ACA had a beneficial effect on reducing some disparities by increasing the number of people covered by health insurance and expanding Medicaid. This is particularly true, she said, regarding access to care and the ability to pay for care. In her opinion, a public health focus and targeting geographical areas with the worst health outcomes is a promising approach to dealing with issues of equity, disparities, and access. Downer offered that funding the services that community health workers deliver in marginalized and underserved communities would make a big difference.

Referring to Slavitt's idea about declaring some aspects of care to be public goods, Chen inquired about some of the principles in identifying

---

[35] For more information, see https://www.congress.gov/bill/116th-congress/senate-bill/829 (accessed May 28, 2019).

aspects of care that would fit in that category and whether such an idea was politically feasible at either the state or federal level. Slavitt replied that aspects of care that affect many people and come with high-cost burdens would be on his list and cited a few examples, such as HIV care and kidney dialysis. In the future, he said, a cure for Alzheimer's disease might fall into the public good category. In his view, it is easier for people to think about specific cases than to have a general rule for what would be a public good. In terms of the political feasibility of this idea, he noted that the best approach might be to work through state attorney generals. Rowland added that one idea regarding insulin is to treat it as a preventive medication that keeps people from ending up in the hospital and include it as part of the preventive services package that is not subject to cost sharing.

Timothy Cox from CareFirst said that his organization increased access by removing the requirement that people must be homebound to qualify for home care, which allows beneficiaries to continue working when possible. CareFirst has also eliminated the 6-month prognosis of death from its eligibility requirements for its hospice and palliative care benefit and allows its members to receive concurrent care.

Machtinger asked if designating treatments such as insulin as public goods would exclude illnesses that are thought to be volitional (such as substance use disorders) but are clearly related to the lived experiences of people who are facing health disparities. Slavitt agreed that this is a hazard and offered one way to address this problem: expand on public sentiment where it exists and influence public sentiment where it does not. In his opinion, mental health and addiction, for example, are less stigmatized today than in the past—in part because the public and politicians are talking about them.

POTENTIAL NEXT STEPS FOR IMPLEMENTING SOLUTIONS TO IMPROVE ACCESS TO CARE AND ACHIEVE HEALTH EQUITY FOR PEOPLE WITH SERIOUS ILLNESS

Shonta Chambers, executive vice president for health equity initiatives and community engagement at the Patient Advocate Foundation, reminded attendees that the workshop was organized around the social ecological model. This model acknowledges there is a role for everyone, from the individual to policy makers, to bring about the culture change needed to achieve health equity and improve access to care for people with serious illness. She asked the panelists in the workshop's final session to reflect on the themes they had heard during the day.

In response, Daniel Dawes, director of the Satcher Health Leadership Institute at the Morehouse School of Medicine and principal investigator and co-founder of the Health Equity Leadership and Exchange Network, highlighted seven themes. First, he noted that health inequities occur throughout life. In Dawes's view, the best solutions to health inequities should involve the most severely affected, employ an ecological approach, leverage peers, ensure access to high-quality communication, and build partnerships at all levels. The health sector by itself, he stressed, cannot address all of the factors that produce health disparities.

Second, patients live in a complex ecosystem in which communities are at the epicenter of health equity. Place and context matter, he pointed out, so communities must be empowered to tackle the multiple intersectional and mutually reinforcing determinants of health inequities.

Third, power, leadership, and relationships are the currency for achieving greater health equity. "Therefore, we all need to work upstream and integrate our approaches to tackling the social, behavioral, and political determinants of health," said Dawes. In addition, it is essential to create or secure the funding mechanisms that can sustain innovative, evidence-based, or promising programs that are advancing health equity.

Fourth, health equity is a moral, cultural, civic, and humanitarian imperative. As a result, it will be necessary to unearth the issues involved and ensure there are interventions in place to address them. Dawes's fifth theme highlighted the need to begin to build the capacity of the workforce in rural, frontier, and urban communities so they understand the role that trauma plays in health care access and delivery. Combining his final two themes, Dawes noted that the health care system has barely changed over the past two decades in terms of accessibility and diversity of clinical trials, for example, or the education medical students receive. In the same way, neither the delivery of care nor the workforce that delivers that care has changed much and is regressing in some respects, particularly in the specialty areas that affect communities of color and other underserved communities. He pointed out that equity is fundamental to quality, and yet there is a dearth of public and private policies prioritizing health equity even with the publication of more than 6,000 peer-reviewed papers on the topic of health equity, minority health, and health disparities. "From a policy standpoint, we have not done enough to move the needle," said Dawes, "and I would really push us to continue focusing on developing and implementing actionable and meaningful policies that utilize an equity lens." What is needed, he posited, are programs, policies, and systems that accommodate a range of beliefs, values, and concerns because a one-size-fits-all approach does not work to address inequities. "Policies impact health, and we have to act," said Dawes.

Finally, he underscored that the pursuit of health equity will be disruptive and uncomfortable. It is threatening, Dawes explained, because the issues that need to be addressed are ingrained in the health care system. While the health care system cannot solve all of the problems that lead to health disparities, it can focus its work and advocacy strategically to tackle these challenges by leveraging the available research.

Steven Clauser, program director, Healthcare Delivery and Disparities Research at PCORI, reiterated the message that evidence-based interventions are available and that research has developed approaches to tailor education for patients and providers. Regarding health care teams, he pointed to the incredible amount of work on the potential key contribution of peer navigators in efforts to increase access and achieve health equity and on the new roles that community health workers can play in educating and improving community health beyond their traditional role of care coordinators, particularly in rural areas.

Technology, said Clauser, can become an important component of the complex intervention packages needed to improve health equity and reduce disparities. Though the role of technology was not discussed at this workshop, he felt it important to note that there will be studies coming out over the next few years that demonstrate how technology will help reduce disparities. Complex intervention packages, he added, seem to have the biggest effect on outcomes. However, complex interventions tend to scare away funders and organizational leaders who have to dedicate resources to enable those interventions and who favor more generic solutions that are sometimes inappropriate for vulnerable populations. Given the diversity of vulnerable populations, it is important to conduct research that compares outcomes associated with interventions that vary in complexity and intensity, and identify which interventions work best for which vulnerable populations and under what circumstances.

Clauser pointed to an area that still needs more research, namely, how to address discrimination. He acknowledged the exciting work that has been done to help train providers to address some of the cultural issues tied to implicit discrimination and added there is research to draw from other areas that have tried to tackle discrimination from a more fundamental perspective. For example, there has been an intentional effort to develop measures of discrimination in the way providers communicate with and treat pregnant women of color or from low-income families. These types of measures could help stimulate quality improvement efforts in organizations committed to reducing health disparities and discrimination.

In her summary of the key messages she heard during the workshop, Barrett stressed the importance of having the patient's voice represented during the workshop. One topic that stood out to her was the conversation around the training of laypeople, patients, community health workers, doctors, nurses, and other members of the care team. Training, said Barrett, has to include fearless conversations that acknowledge both the historical and current experiences that most marginalized and vulnerable populations deal with throughout their lives. She noted there are a number of available trainings around implicit bias, but it is unclear what works and what knowledge and skills people need so as to engage in interactions with patients in a way that minimizes or eliminates implicit bias. Culturally sensitive or responsive communication training is another area where more work could be done, particularly around conversations that identify the goals of a patient with serious illness and that build trust with the patient.

Barrett also highlighted the importance of leveraging partnerships in the work to increase access to care and achieve health equity and commented on the need to look for partners beyond the usual ones. In her view, it is important to look for more innovative organizations, particularly those in the community, to engage in such efforts on a regular basis. Implementation of evidence-based interventions is also an area that both needs more research and could be developed through strategic partnerships. Barrett added that quality improvement measures should be implemented using a health equity lens. Ultimately, she said, improving patient and population level outcomes must be the end goal of any intervention.

The final panelist, Maguire, remarked that in her view, it was clear from Bridgette Hempstead's story presented in the opening session that there has been little progress on access and equity over the past two decades, a situation that she said is unacceptable and requires an urgent response. Referencing what other speakers throughout the day stated, Maguire reiterated that there is no one solution for every person and every community, making it imperative that any solution is developed with community input. Maguire emphasized that building trust with community members is essential and that this process starts with health care professionals taking personal responsibility for recognizing their individual biases and backgrounds and how these present in conversations with patients and community members.

Maguire emphasized that palliative care can be an effective intervention to reduce health disparities. Her organization offers a health plan benefit that has included palliative care since 2014, but the uptake of this benefit has not been as robust as expected. As result, more work is necessary to educate clients in the Blue Cross and Blue Shield network about palliative care, according to Maguire. She noted that her organization is developing metrics and financial incentives to measure and reward quality and equity in value-based payment arrangements. In Maguire's view, payers have the ability to influence the social determinants of health and see that they are addressed by provider organizations. She also encouraged consideration of how health systems exert influence over awareness of the social determinants of health.

Maguire said that workforce development was a challenge, starting with how clinicians are educated to be compassionate and treat the whole person (as opposed to treating a person as a vessel of disease). Maguire commented she was struck by the lack of diversity in the clinician population, with few physicians being people of color, as Johnson had highlighted in her presentation. "We need to think systematically about how to change that number," she said. It is also important to continue thinking about how to foster a more diverse, team-based approach through education and training that includes community health workers, said Maguire. Her final comment was on the importance of tailoring ACP so that it is appropriate to the individual and their community.

Potential Next Steps to Advance Access and Equity

Upon prompting from Chambers, the panelists discussed the actionable steps they would recommend based on their experiences and the day's discussions. Maguire proposed investing in workforce and leadership development. Her organization, for example, has been funding programs in both areas, and its Sojourns Scholars Leadership Program[36] invests in 12 emerging leaders in palliative care annually. The foundation's hope, she explained, is that these Sojourns Scholars will create a critical mass of leaders who will influence not only serious illness care but health care delivery in general. She noted that Sanders, who spoke in the third session, is a Sojourns Scholar, and a number of his fellow scholars are working on health disparities issues, mostly through a communication lens.

Barrett described how she started the Duke Cancer Institute's Office of Health Equity. She explained how she, together with her colleagues,

---

[36] For more information, see https://www.cambiahealthfoundation.org/funding-areas/sojourns-scholars-leadership-program.html (accessed May 10, 2019).

community leaders, and stakeholders, spent nearly 1 year conducting focus groups with the broader community, patients, caregivers, health departments, research teams, and the institution's leadership to find out what her office would mean to those who would use it and what resources it could provide to patients and community members. Afterward, she, along with community partners, reported back to more than 300 people who came to a community event and discussed her office's strategic plan, which included creating a community advisory council of 23 representatives from the various communities served by the Duke Cancer Institute.

One feature of her office's efforts is community-facing navigation that relies on community health workers to deliver evidence-based approaches for increasing access to quality care and advance health equity. This effort has been successful because it leverages trusted members of the community who understand the nuances of the local culture when working with individuals. A second area of emphasis has been to identify opportunities to increase the diversity of clinical trial participants, and a third identifies ways of diversifying her organization's workforce. She has also created a program called Just Ask: Diversity in Clinical Research Training Program[37] that helps research teams and coordinators understand how implicit bias and sociocultural norms and perspectives can affect how they communicate with potential and current research participants, and how to develop strategies to address them.

Clauser suggested involving patients and key stakeholders in whatever work one is doing, particularly when planning and conducting research. His organization requires that researchers involve patients, clinicians, health care leaders, and payers in all phases of the study, from designing the study and selecting outcomes measures, monitoring trial operations, and reviewing the study's final results. This level of involvement, he said, often comes with an obligation for implementation. In one instance, he and his colleagues decided to bring together stakeholders to discuss ongoing research related to studies of community health workers with the goal of possibly making adjustments or adding more data elements that would make the results more relevant to the stakeholders' communities. The discussions between patients and payers about relevant outcomes and process measures produced ideas that will enhance some ongoing studies and will influence the next generation of research projects that PCORI will undertake. Clauser noted

---

[37] For more information, see http://dukecancerinstitute.org/news/diversity-training-pilot-research-teams-launched (accessed May 24, 2019).

that PCORI's palliative care initiative was certainly influenced by this type of patient and stakeholder input.

Dawes approached the problem from the perspective of the political determinants of health and public policies' significant effect on the ability to achieve health equity. He and his collaborators at the Health Equity Leadership & Exchange Network are pushing for more equitable policies to counteract a trend he has seen where courts are increasingly determining that discrimination in health care is a social issue, not a legal one. What this interpretation means from a legal perspective, according to Dawes, is that there is no constitutional basis for remedying discrimination and disparities in health. In his opinion, the political determinants of health are inaccurately portrayed as social determinants.

Dawes also stressed the need to increase the diversity of the predomi-nantly White workforce to serve a much more diverse patient population, and he highlighted the woefully inadequate enrollment of Black men in medical school. "This never-ending battle for health equity requires not only a dedicated and culturally competent roster of health equity champions but … a diverse clinical and allied health workforce that includes the commu-nity health workers as a key partner," said Dawes. "They are the bridge into the communities." Tying this back to the policy world, he said that the push for diversification of the clinical workforce is not only an admirable cause to champion but essential to support every other health policy. For example, he noted that the predominantly African American communities in rural Georgia are extremely mistrustful of the health care system, but when those communities see health workers who look like them, they are more likely to agree to preventive services.

Leveraging Connections and Developing Partnerships

The last question Chambers posed to the panelists was to identify one specific action that could be taken at any level of the spheres in the social ecological model that would benefit the individual at the center of that model. Maguire's suggestion was to use community health workers (CHWs) and places of worship to encourage ACP across all populations. Dawes and Clauser both expressed a desire to mobilize individuals to tell their com-pelling stories to policy makers to emphasize the importance of increasing access to care and reducing health inequities. Clauser noted that the per-sonal stories told during the workshop were the most powerful parts of the day, and he recounted how personal stories about the benefits of telehealth for individuals with Parkinson's disease contributed to PCORI's decision to fund a follow-on implementation and dissemination study that involves the American Neurological Association in the creation of a telehealth therapy training program.[38]

Barrett proposed expanding the partnerships with community health workers to develop a trustworthy space for patients in marginalized and underrepresented communities. She noted in particular a PCORI-funded study that is looking at how community health workers have the potential to increase ACP among African Americans, with the goal of reducing the disparity between Blacks and Whites. She pointed out that it represents a great opportunity to think about how to address health equity and end-of-life decisions in underserved communities by engaging CHWs from the local community. An important contributor to getting this study off the ground, she said, was involving stakeholders and community health workers early in its development and the effect their personal stories had on the investigators and each other. "Storytelling is so important for advocacy, but it is also important for the work we are doing right now in terms of simply getting people access to the care they need," explained Barrett. She stressed the importance of "making sure that we create a trustworthy space for community health workers and other stakeholders to tell their stories and be key players in helping to move the work forward." Dawes quoted his friend, mentor, and former Surgeon General, David Satcher: "In order to eliminate disparities in health and achieve health equity, we need leaders who care enough, know enough, have the courage to do enough and who will persevere until the job is done."

Closing Remarks

Chambers concluded the workshop by stating, "We may not have all the answers, but we have the opportunity to do something. If we have the passion, drive, and determination to disrupt the status quo and realize that ensuring equity goes beyond equality and must be positioned as an urgent social justice issue, then we all play a part in activating and advancing solutions."

---

[38] For more information, see https://www.pcori.org/research-results/2013/do-video-house-calls-specialist-help-get-care-people-parkinsons-disease (accessed July 11, 2019).

REFERENCES

Alexander, R., K. Parker, and T. Schwetz. 2016. Sexual and gender minority health research at the National Institutes of Health. *LGBT Health* 3(1):7–10.

Bauer, L. 2018. Reducing food insecurity among households with children is still a challenge for the United States. https://www.brookings.edu/blog/up-front/2018/07/25/reducing-food-insecurity-among-households-with-children-is-still-a-challenge-for-the-united-states (accessed May 30, 2019).

Boccuti, C., G. Jacobson, K. Orgera, and T. Neuman. 2018. *Medigap enrollment and consumer protections vary across states.* Henry J. Kaiser Family Foundation. http://files.kff.org/attachment/Issue-Brief-Medigap-Enrollment-and-Consumer-Protections-Vary-Across-States (accessed August 13, 2019).

Boehmer, U., X. Miao, and A. Ozonoff. 2011. Cancer survivorship and sexual orientation. *Cancer* 117(16):3796–3804.

Brooks, T., L. Roygardner, and S. Artiga. 2019. *Medicaid and CHIP eligibility, enrollment, and cost sharing policies as of January 2019: Findings from a 50-state survey.* Henry J. Kaiser Family Foundation. http://files.kff.org/attachment/Report-Medicaid-and-CHIP-Eligibility-Enrollment-Renewal-and-Cost-Sharing-Policies-as-of-January-2019 (accessed August 13, 2019).

Brotman, S., B. Ryan, and R. Cormier. 2003. The health and social service needs of gay and lesbian elders and their families in Canada. *Gerontologist* 43(2):192–202.

Burke, S. E., J. F. Dovidio, J. M. Przedworski, R. R. Hardeman, S. P. Perry, S. M. Phelan, D. B. Nelson, D. J. Burgess, M. W. Yeazel, and M. van Ryn. 2015. Do contact and empathy mitigate bias against gay and lesbian people among heterosexual first-year medical students? A report from the Medical Student Change Study. *Academic Medicine: Journal of the Association of American Medical Colleges* 90(5):645–651.

California Health Care Foundation. 2019. *Medi-Cal.* https://www.chcf.org/topic/medi-cal (accessed May 21, 2019).

CAPC (Center to Advance Palliative Care). 2015. *America's care of serious illness: 2015 state-by-state report card on access to palliative care in our nation's hospitals.* https://reportcard.capc.org/wp-content/uploads/2015/08/CAPC-Report-Card-2015.pdf (accessed August 13, 2019).

CDC (Centers for Disease Control and Prevention). 2011. *Social ecological model.* https://www.cdc.gov/violenceprevention/publichealthissue/social-ecologicalmodel.html (accessed August 19, 2019).

CDC. 2018. *Suicides among American Indian/Alaska Natives—national violent death reporting system, 18 states, 2003–2014.* https://www.cdc.gov/mmwr/volumes/67/wr/mm6708a1.htm (accessed August 19, 2019).

CDC. 2019a. *Adverse childhood experiences (ACEs).* https://www.cdc.gov/violenceprevention/childabuseandneglect/acestudy/index.html?CDC_AA_refVal=https%3A%2F%2Fwww.cdc.gov%2Fviolenceprevention%2Facestudy%2Findex.html (accessed May 21, 2019).

CDC. 2019b. *Burden of tobacco use in the U.S.: Current cigarette smoking among U.S. adults aged 18 years and older.* https://www.cdc.gov/tobacco/campaign/tips/resources/data/cigarette-smoking-in-united-states.html#three (accessed May 28, 2019).

CDC. 2019c. *HIV among African Americans.* https://www.cdc.gov/nchhstp/newsroom/docs/factsheets/cdc-hiv-aa-508.pdf (accessed May 21, 2019).

CDC. 2019d. *HIV and transgender people.* https://www.cdc.gov/hiv/group/gender/transgender/index.html (accessed May 28, 2019).

CDC. 2019e. *Pregnancy-related deaths.* https://www.cdc.gov/reproductivehealth/maternalinfanthealth/pregnancy-relatedmortality.htm (accessed May 21, 2019).

CDC NCCDPHP (National Center for Chronic Disease Prevention and Health Promotion). 2016. *Collaborating with community health workers to enhance the coordination of care and advance health equity.* https://www.cdc.gov/nccdphp/dch/pdfs/dch-chw-issue-brief.pdf (accessed August 19, 2019).

Chen, A. H. M. 2019. A view from the safety net: San Francisco Health Network (paper presented at Improving Access to and Equity of Care for People with Serious Illness: A Workshop, Washington, DC, April 4, 2019).

Chin, M. H. 2014. How to achieve health equity. *New England Journal of Medicine* 371(24):2331–2332.

Chin, M. H., A. R. Clarke, R. S. Nocon, A. A. Casey, A. P. Goddu, N. M. Keesecker, and S. C. Cook. 2012. A roadmap and best practices for organizations to reduce racial and ethnic disparities in health care. *Journal of General Internal Medicine* 27(8):992–1000.

Cierra Sisters. 2019. *Cierra Sisters.* http://www.cierrasisters.org (accessed May 21, 2019).

Clarke, A. R., O. L. Vargas, A. P. Goddu, K. W. McCullough, R. DeMeester, S. C. Cook, M. El-Shamaa, and M. H. Chin. 2012. *A roadmap to reduce racial and ethnic disparities in health care.* Princeton, NJ: Robert Wood Johnson Foundation.

Cooper, L. A., D. L. Roter, R. L. Johnson, D. E. Ford, D. M. Steinwachs, and N. R. Powe. 2003. Patient-centered communication, ratings of care, and concordance of patient and physician race. *Annals of Internal Medicine* 139(11):907–915.

Cronholm, P. F., C. M. Forke, R. Wade, M. H. Bair-Merritt, M. Davis, M. Harkins-Schwarz, L. M. Pachter, and J. A. Fein. 2015. Adverse childhood experiences: Expanding the concept of adversity. *American Journal of Preventive Medicine* 49(3):354–361.

Cubanski, J., T. Neuman, K. Orgera, and A. Damico. 2017. *No limit: Medicare Part D enrollees exposed to high out-of-pocket drug costs without a hard cap on spending.* Henry J. Kaiser Family Foundation. http://files.kff.org/attachment/Issue-Brief-No-Limit-Medicare-Part-D-Enrollees-Exposed-to-High-Out-of-Pocket-Drug-Costs-Without-a-Hard-Cap-on-Spending (accessed August 13, 2019).

Cubanski, J., A. Damico, T. Neuman, and G. Jacobson. 2018a. *Sources of supplemental coverage among Medicare beneficiaries in 2016.* Henry J. Kaiser Family Foundation. https://www.kff.org/medicare/issue-brief/sources-of-supplemental-coverage-among-medicare-beneficiaries-in-2016 (accessed August 13, 2019).

Cubanski, J., T. Neuman, and A. Damico. 2018b. *Closing the Medicare Part D coverage gap: Trends, recent changes, and what's ahead.* Henry J. Kaiser Family Foundation. https://www.kff.org/medicare/issue-brief/closing-the-medicare-part-d-coverage-gap-trends-recent-changes-and-whats-ahead (accessed August 13, 2019).

Cubanski, J., W. Koma, and T. Neuman. 2019. *The out-of-pocket cost burden for specialty drugs in Medicare Part D in 2019.* Henry J. Kaiser Family Foundation. https://www.kff.org/medicare/issue-brief/the-out-of-pocket-cost-burden-for-specialty-drugs-in-medicare-part-d-in-2019 (accessed August 13, 2019).

Dandapani, S. V., M. Eaton, C. R. Thomas, Jr., and P. G. Pagnini. 2010. HIV-positive anal cancer: An update for the clinician. *Journal of Gastrointestinal Oncology* 1(1):34–44.

Deni, H. 2012. *Finding pride in caring: LGBT caregivers answer the call from the community.* https://www.asaging.org/blog/finding-pride-caring-lgbt-caregivers-answer-call-community (accessed July 8, 2019).

Dibble, S. L., S. A. Roberts, and B. Nussey. 2004. Comparing breast cancer risk between lesbians and their heterosexual sisters. *Women's Health Issues* 14(2):60–68.

Durso, L. E., and I. H. Meyer. 2013. Patterns and predictors of disclosure of sexual orientation to healthcare providers among lesbians, gay men, and bisexuals. *Sexuality Research & Social Policy* 10(1):35–42.

Eiken, S., K. Sredl, B. Burwell, and A. Amos. 2018. *Medicaid expenditures for long-term services and supports in FY 2016.* https://www.medicaid.gov/medicaid/ltss/downloads/reports-and-evaluations/ltssexpenditures2016.pdf (accessed August 13, 2019).

Feeding America. 2019. *What is food insecurity?* https://hungerandhealth.feedingamerica.org/understand-food-insecurity (accessed May 30, 2019).

Felitti, V. J., R. F. Anda, D. Nordenberg, D. F. Williamson, A. M. Spitz, V. Edwards, M. P. Koss, and J. S. Marks. 1998. Relationship of childhood abuse and household dysfunction to many of the leading causes of death in adults. The Adverse Childhood Experiences (ACE) study. *American Journal of Preventive Medicine* 14(4):245–258.

Garcia, M. 2014. Study: Antigay communities lead to early LGB death. *Advocate*, February 16.

Garfield, G., K. Orgera, and A. Damico. 2019. *The uninsured and the ACA: A primer—key facts about health insurance and the uninsured amidst changes to the Affordable Care Act.* Henry J. Kaiser Family Foundation. https://www.kff.org/uninsured/report/the-uninsured-and-the-aca-a-primer-key-facts-about-health-insurance-and-the-uninsured-amidst-changes-to-the-affordable-care-act (accessed August 13, 2019).

Gates, G. J. 2014. *In U.S., LGBT more likely than non-LGBT to be uninsured.* Washington, DC: Gallup.

Gilligan, A. M., D. S. Alberts, D. J. Roe, and G. H. Skrepnek. 2018. Death or debt? National estimates of financial toxicity in persons with newly diagnosed cancer. *American Journal of Medicine* 131(10):1187–1199.

Goepp, J. G., S. Meykler, N. E. Mooney, C. Lyon, R. Raso, and K. Julliard. 2008. Provider insights about palliative care barriers and facilitators: Results of a rapid ethnographic assessment. *American Journal of Hospice and Palliative Care* 25(4):309–314.

Gordon, H. S., R. L. Street, Jr., B. F. Sharf, P. A. Kelly, and J. Souchek. 2006. Racial differences in trust and lung cancer patients' perceptions of physician communication. *Journal of Clinical Oncology* 24(6):904–909.

Gorn, D. 2018. Food for the heart in a new California health program. *CALmatters News.* https://calmatters.org/health/2018/07/food-for-the-heart-in-a-new-california-health-program (accessed August 13, 2019).

GovTrack.us. 2019. *S. 2786—114th Congress: Rural Access to Hospice Act of 2016.* https://www.govtrack.us/congress/bills/114/s2786 (accessed May 29, 2019).

Grant, J. M., L. A. Mottet, J. Tanis, J. Harrison, J. L. Herman, and M. Keisling. 2011. *Injustice at every turn: A report of the National Transgender Discrimination Survey.* Washington, DC. https://www.transequality.org/sites/default/files/docs/resources/NTDS_Report.pdf (accessed August 13, 2019).

Gunja, M. Z., R. Tikkanen, S. Seervai, and S. R. Collins. 2018. *What is the status of women's health and health care in the U.S. compared to ten other countries?* The Commonwealth Fund. https://www.commonwealthfund.org/publications/issue-briefs/2018/dec/womens-health-us-compared-ten-other-countries (accessed August 13, 2019).

Haider, A. H., E. B. Schneider, L. M. Kodadek, R. R. Adler, A. Ranjit, M. Torain, R. Y. Shields, C. Snyder, J. D. Schuur, L. Vail, D. German, S. Peterson, and B. D. Lau. 2017. Emergency department query for patient-centered approaches to sexual orientation and gender identity: The equality study. *JAMA Internal Medicine* 177(6):819–828.

Harris Interactive. 2005. *New national survey shows financial concerns and lack of adequate health insurance are top causes for delay by lesbians in obtaining health care.* http://marketresearchworld.net/content/view/276/77 (accessed May 30, 2019).

Hart, T. L., D. W. Coon, M. A. Kowalkowski, K. Zhang, J. I. Hersom, H. H. Goltz, D. A. Wittmann, and D. M. Latini. 2014. Changes in sexual roles and quality of life for gay men after prostate cancer: Challenges for sexual health providers. *The Journal of Sexual Medicine* 11(9):2308–2317.

Hatzenbuehler, M. L., K. M. Keyes, and D. S. Hasin. 2009. State-level policies and psychiatric morbidity in lesbian, gay, and bisexual populations. *American Journal of Public Health* 99(12):2275–2281.

Hempstead, B., C. Green, K. J. Briant, B. Thompson, and Y. Molina. 2018. Community Empowerment Partners (CEPs): A breast health education program for African-American women. *Journal of Community Health* 43(5):833–841.

Herman, J. L. 2013. Gendered restrooms and minority stress: The public regulation of gender and its impact on transgender people's lives. *Journal of Public Management and Social Policy* 19(1):65–80.

HHS (Department of Health and Human Services) Administration Bureau of Health Professions. 2016. *Supporting diversity in the health professions.* https://www.hrsa.gov/advisorycommittees/bhpradvisory/cogme/Publications/diversityresourcepaper.pdf (accessed August 13, 2019).

HHS Office of Minority Health. 2017. *Infant mortality and African Americans.* https://minorityhealth.hhs.gov/omh/browse.aspx?lvl=4&lvlid=23 (accessed May 21, 2019).

Hoffman, K. M., S. Trawalter, J. R. Axt, and M. N. Oliver. 2016. Racial bias in pain assessment and treatment recommendations, and false beliefs about biological differences between blacks and whites. *Proceedings of the National Academy of Sciences of the United States of America* 113(16):4296–4301.

IOM (Institute of Medicine). 2001. *Crossing the quality chasm: A new health system for the 21st century.* Washington, DC: National Academy Press.

IOM. 2013a. *Delivering high-quality cancer care: Charting a new course for a system in crisis.* Washington, DC: The National Academies Press.

IOM. 2013b. *Collecting sexual orientation and gender identity data in electronic health records: Workshop summary.* Washington, DC: The National Academies Press.

IOM. 2015. *Dying in America: Improving quality and honoring individual preferences near the end of life.* Washington, DC: The National Academies Press.

Irving, M. 2019. *Health Partners Plans executives volunteer in MANNA's Kitchen.* https://www.healthpartnersplans.com/about-us/newsroom/news-releases/2019/health-partners-plans-executives-volunteer-in-manna-s-kitchen (accessed August 13, 2019).

Johnson, K. S. 2013. Racial and ethnic disparities in palliative care. *Journal of Palliative Medicine* 16(11):1329–1334.

Kaiser Family Foundation. 2017. *Percent of private sector establishments that offer health insurance to employees.* https://www.kff.org/other/state-indicator/percent-of-firms-offering-coverage/?currentTimeframe=0&sortModel=%7B%22colId%22:%22Location%22,%22sort%22:%22asc%22%7D (accessed August 13, 2019).

Kaiser Family Foundation. 2018a. *Medicaid in the United States.* http://files.kff.org/attachment/fact-sheet-medicaid-state-US (accessed August 13, 2019).

Kaiser Family Foundation. 2018b. *An overview of the Medicare Part D prescription drug benefit.* https://www.kff.org/medicare/fact-sheet/an-overview-of-the-medicare-part-d-prescription-drug-benefit (accessed August 13, 2019).

Kaiser Family Foundation. 2019a. *Medicaid managed care market tracker.* https://www.kff.org/data-collection/medicaid-managed-care-market-tracker (accessed May 21, 2019).

Kaiser Family Foundation. 2019b. *Status of state Medicaid expansion decisions: Interactive map.* https://www.kff.org/medicaid/issue-brief/status-of-state-medicaid-expansion-decisions-interactive-map (accessed May 21, 2019).

Kaiser Family Foundation. 2019c. *Where are states today? Medicaid and CHIP eligibility levels for children, pregnant women, and adults.* https://www.kff.org/medicaid/fact-sheet/where-are-states-today-medicaid-and-chip (accessed August 13, 2019).

Kamal, A. H., J. H. Bull, K. M. Swetz, S. P. Wolf, T. D. Shanafelt, and E. R. Myers. 2017. Future of the palliative care workforce: Preview to an impending crisis. *The American Journal of Medicine* 130(2):113–114.

Kamen, C., K. M. Mustian, A. Dozier, D. J. Bowen, and Y. Li. 2015a. Disparities in psychological distress impacting lesbian, gay, bisexual and transgender cancer survivors. *Psycho-Oncology* 24(11):1384–1391.

Kamen, C. S., M. Smith-Stoner, C. E. Heckler, M. Flannery, and L. Margolies. 2015b. Social support, self-rated health, and lesbian, gay, bisexual, and transgender identity disclosure to cancer care providers. *Oncology Nursing Forum* 42(1):44–51.

Katz, A. 2009. Gay and lesbian patients with cancer. *Oncology Nursing Forum* 36(2):203–207.

Kauffman, J. 2017. City's health care initiative shows success, but questions remain. *San Francisco Chronicle*, October 24.

Khullar, D., and D. A. Chokshi. 2018. *Health, income, and poverty: Where we are and what could help.* Princeton, NJ: Health Affairs, Robert Wood Johnson Foundation.

Kirzinger, A., L. Lopes, B. We, and M. Brodie. 2019. *KFF health tracking poll—February 2019: Prescription drugs.* https://www.kff.org/health-costs/poll-finding/kff-health-tracking-poll-february-2019-prescription-drugs (accessed May 9, 2019).

Levin, B., J. J. Nolan, and J. D. Reitzel. 2018. *New data shows US hate crimes continued to rise in 2017.* http://theconversation.com/new-data-shows-us-hate-crimes-continued-to-rise-in-2017-97989 (accessed June 7, 2019).

Lim, F., A., M. Johnson, and M. Eliason. 2015. A national survey of faculty knowledge, experience, and readiness for teaching lesbian, gay, bisexual and transgender health in baccalaureate nursing programs. *Nursing Education Perspectives* 36(3):144–152.

Loggers, E. T., P. K. Maciejewski, E. Paulk, S. DeSanto-Madeya, M. Nilsson, K. Viswanath, A. A. Wright, T. A. Balboni, J. Temel, H. Stieglitz, S. Block, and H. G. Prigerson. 2009. Racial differences in predictors of intensive end-of-life care in patients with advanced cancer. *Journal of Clinical Oncology* 27(33):5559–5564.

Machtinger, E. L., Y. P. Cuca, N. Khanna, C. D. Rose, and L. S. Kimberg. 2015a. From treatment to healing: The promise of trauma-informed primary care. *Women's Health Issues* 25(3):193–197.

Machtinger, E. L., S. M. Lavin, S. Hilliard, R. Jones, J. E. Haberer, K. Capito, and C. Dawson-Rose. 2015b. An expressive therapy group disclosure intervention for women living with HIV improves social support, self-efficacy, and the safety and quality of relationships: A qualitative analysis. *The Journal of the Association of Nurses in AIDS Care* 26(2):187–198.

Machtinger, E. L., K. B. Davis, L. S. Kimberg, N. Khanna, Y. P. Cuca, C. Dawson-Rose, M. Shumway, J. Campbell, A. Lewis-O'Connor, M. Blake, A. Blanch, and B. McCaw. 2019. From treatment to healing: Inquiry and response to recent and past trauma in adult health care. *Women's Health Issues* 29(2):97–102.

Mack, J. W., M. E. Paulk, K. Viswanath, and H. G. Prigerson. 2010. Racial disparities in the outcomes of communication on medical care received near death. *Archives of Internal Medicine* 170(17):1533–1540.

Margolies, L., and N. Scout. 2013. *LGBT patient-centered outcomes: Cancer survivors teach us how to improve care for all.* https://cancer-network.org/wp-content/uploads/2017/02/lgbt-patient-centered-outcomes.pdf (accessed May 29, 2019).

McLaughlin, S. 2010. Traditions and diabetes prevention: A healthy path for Native Americans. *Diabetes Spectrum* 23(4):272–277.

MedPAC (Medicare Payment Advisory Commission). 2004. *Chapter 6: Hospice care in Medicare: Recent trends and a review of the issues (June 2004 report).* http://67.59.137.244/publications/congressional_reports/June04_ch6.pdf (accessed August 13, 2019).

MedPAC. 2011. *Chapter 11: Hospice (March 2011 report).* http://medpac.gov/docs/default-source/reports/Mar11_EntireReport.pdf (accessed August 13, 2019).

MedPAC. 2012. *Chapter 11: Hospice services (March 2012 report).* http://www.medpac.gov/docs/default-source/reports/chapter-11-hospice-services-march-2012-report-.pdf?sfvrsn=0 (accessed August 13, 2019).

MedPAC. 2013. *Chapter 12: Hospice services (March 2013 report).* http://www.medpac.gov/docs/default-source/reports/mar13_medpac_ch12.pdf?sfvrsn=0 (accessed August 13, 2019).

MedPAC. 2014. *Chapter 12: Hospice services (March 2014 report).* http://www.medpac.gov/docs/default-source/reports/mar14_medpac_ch12.pdf?sfvrsn=0 (accessed August 13, 2019).

MedPAC. 2015. *Chapter 12: Hospice services (March 2015 report).* http://www.medpac.gov/docs/default-source/reports/mar15_medpac_ch12.pdf?sfvrsn=0 (accessed August 13, 2019).

MedPAC. 2016. *Chapter 12: Hospice services (March 2016 report).* http://www.medpac.gov/docs/default-source/reports/mar16_medpac_ch12.pdf?sfvrsn=0 (accessed August 13, 2019).

MedPAC. 2017. *Chapter 12: Hospice services (March 2017 report).* http://www.medpac.gov/docs/default-source/reports/mar17_medpac_ch12.pdf?sfvrsn=0 (accessed August 13, 2019).

MedPAC. 2018. *Chapter 12: Hospice services (March 2018 report).* http://www.medpac.gov/docs/default-source/reports/mar18_medpac_ch12_sec.pdf?sfvrsn=0 (accessed August 13, 2019).

Meghani, S. H., E. Byun, and R. M. Gallagher. 2012. Time to take stock: A meta-analysis and systematic review of analgesic treatment disparities for pain in the United States. *Pain Medicine* 13(2):150–174.

Missourians to End Poverty. 2018. *2018 Missouri poverty report.* Jefferson City, MO. http://www.caastlc.org/wpsite/wp-content/uploads/2018/03/MCAN-MEP-2018-MissouriPovertyReport-DigitalDownload.pdf (accessed August 13, 2019).

Musumeci, M., and M. O. Watts. 2019. *Key state policy choices about Medicaid home and community-based services.* Henry J. Kaiser Family Foundation. https://www.kff.org/medicaid/issue-brief/key-state-policy-choices-about-medicaid-home-and-community-based-services (accessed August 13, 2019).

Musumeci, M., P. Chidambaram, and M. O. Watts. 2016. *Medicaid financial eligibility for seniors and people with disabilities: Findings from a 50-state survey.* Henry J. Kaiser Family Foundation. https://www.kff.org/medicaid/issue-brief/medicaid-financial-eligibility-for-seniors-and-people-with-disabilities-findings-from-a-50-state-survey (accessed August 13, 2019).

Musumeci, M., P. Chidambaram, and M. O. Watts. 2019a. *Key questions about Medicaid home and community-based services waiver waiting lists.* Henry J. Kaiser Family Foundation. https://www.kff.org/medicaid/issue-brief/key-questions-about-medicaid-home-and-community-based-services-waiver-waiting-lists (accessed August 13, 2019).

Musumeci, M., P. Chidambaram, and M. O. Watts. 2019b. *Medicaid home and community-based services enrollment and spending.* Henry J. Kaiser Family Foundation. https://www.kff.org/medicaid/issue-brief/medicaid-home-and-community-based-services-enrollment-and-spending (accessed August 13, 2019).

NASEM (National Academies of Sciences, Engineering, and Medicine). 2018. *Making medicines affordable: A national imperative.* Washington, DC: The National Academies Press.

NCI (National Cancer Institute). 2015. *SEER cancer statistics review 1975–2012.* Bethesda, MD: National Cancer Institute.

NHPCO (National Hospice and Palliative Care Organization) HAN (Hospice Action Network). 2017. *Rural Access to Hospice Act.* http://hospiceactionnetwork.org/linked_documents/get_informed/legislation/2018%20Rural%20Update.pdf (accessed May 21, 2019).

NIH (National Institutes of Health) Sexual and Gender Minority Research Coordinating Committee. 2015. *NIH FY 2016–2020 strategic plan to advance research on the health and well-being of sexual and gender minorities.* Bethesda, MD: National Institutes of Health.

NQF (National Quality Forum). 2017. A roadmap for promoting health equity and eliminating disparities: The four I's for health equity. Washington, DC: National Quality Forum.

Obedin-Maliver, J., E. S. Goldsmith, L. Stewart, W. White, E. Tran, S. Brenman, M. Wells, D. M. Fetterman, G. Garcia, and M. R. Lunn. 2011. Lesbian, gay, bisexual, and transgender–related content in undergraduate medical education. *JAMA* 306(9):971–977.

Palar, K., T. Napoles, L. L. Hufstedler, H. Seligman, F. M. Hecht, K. Madsen, M. Ryle, S. Pitchford, E. A. Frongillo, and S. D. Weiser. 2017. Comprehensive and medically appropriate food support is associated with improved HIV and diabetes health. *Journal of Urban Health: Bulletin of the New York Academy of Medicine* 94(1):87–99.

Park, H., and I. Mykhyalyshyn. 2016. LGBT people are more likely to be targets of hate crimes than any other minority group. *The New York Times*, June 16.

Pathela, P., A. Hajat, J. Schillinger, S. Blank, R. Sell, and F. Mostashari. 2006. Discordance between sexual behavior and self-reported sexual identity: A population-based survey of New York City men. *Annals of Internal Medicine* 145(6):416–425.

Penner, L. A., I. V. Blair, T. L. Albrecht, and J. F. Dovidio. 2014. Reducing racial health care disparities: A social psychological analysis. *Policy Insights from the Behavioral and Brain Sciences* 1(1):204–212.

Periyakoil, V. S., E. Neri, and H. Kraemer. 2015. No easy talk: A mixed methods study of doctor reported barriers to conducting effective end-of-life conversations with diverse patients. *PLoS ONE* 10(4):e0122321.

Rhodes, R. L., J. M. Teno, and S. R. Connor. 2007. African American bereaved family members' perceptions of the quality of hospice care: Lessened disparities, but opportunities to improve remain. *Journal of Pain and Symptom Management* 34(5):472–479.

Roeder, A. 2019. America is failing its black mothers. *Harvard Public Health: Magazine of the Harvard T.H. Chan School of Public Health.* https://www.hsph.harvard.edu/magazine/magazine_article/america-is-failing-its-black-mothers (accessed August 13, 2019).

Rosenberg, E. S., G. A. Millett, P. S. Sullivan, C. Del Rio, and J. W. Curran. 2014. Understanding the HIV disparities between black and white men who have sex with men in the USA using the HIV care continuum: A modeling study. *The Lancet HIV* 1(3):e112–e118.

RWJF (Robert Wood Johnson Foundation). 2019. *Childhood obesity trends.* https://www.stateofobesity.org/childhood-obesity-trends (accessed May 21, 2019).

Sabin, J. A., R. G. Riskind, and B. A. Nosek. 2015. Health care providers' implicit and explicit attitudes toward lesbian women and gay men. *American Journal of Public Health* 105(9):1831–1841.

SAMHSA (Substance Abuse and Mental Health Services Administration). 2014. *SAMHSA's concept of trauma and guidance for a trauma-informed approach.* HHS Publication No. (SMA) 14-4884 SAMSHA. https://store.samhsa.gov/file/23565/download?token=GOhI_HdC (accessed August 13, 2019).

Sanders, J. J., M. T. Robinson, and S. D. Block. 2016. Factors impacting advance care planning among African Americans: Results of a systematic integrated review. *Journal of Palliative Medicine* 19(2):202–227.

Sanders, J. J., J. R. Curtis, and J. A. Tulsky. 2018. Achieving goal-concordant care: A conceptual model and approach to measuring serious illness communication and its impact. *Journal of Palliative Medicine* 21(S2):S17–S27.

Sanders, J. J., K. S. Johnson, K. Cannady, J. Paladino, D. W. Ford, S. D. Block, and K. R. Sterba. 2019. From barriers to assets: Rethinking factors impacting advance care planning for African Americans. *Palliative and Supportive Care* 17(3):306–313.

Sharma, R. K., K. A. Cameron, J. S. Chmiel, J. H. Von Roenn, E. Szmuilowicz, H. G. Prigerson, and F. J. Penedo. 2015. Racial/ethnic differences in inpatient palliative care consultation for patients with advanced cancer. *Journal of Clinical Oncology* 33(32):3802–3808.

Shierholz, H. 2013. *Low wages and scant benefits leave many in-home workers unable to make ends meet.* Economy Policy Institute. https://www.epi.org/publication/in-home-workers (accessed August 13, 2019).

Smith, C., P. Prioleau, M. Zhang, A. Wajnberg, and K. Ornstein. 2015. Palliative care outcomes of minority patients receiving home-based primary and palliative care (FR436-A). *Journal of Pain and Symptom Management* 49(2):368.

The Commonwealth Fund. 2008. Survey: 79 million Americans have problems with medical bills or debt. *The Commonwealth Fund Newsletter.* https://www.commonwealthfund.org/publications/newsletter-article/survey-79-million-americans-have-problems-medical-bills-or-debt (accessed August 13, 2019).

U.S. Census Bureau. 2017. Poverty status in the past 12 months by sex and age. *American Community Survey 5-year estimates.* U.S. Census Bureau. https://www.census.gov/programs-surveys/acs/news/data-releases/2017/release.html (accessed August 13, 2019).

Wade, R., Jr., P. F. Cronholm, J. A. Fein, C. M. Forke, M. B. Davis, M. Harkins-Schwarz, L. M. Pachter, and M. H. Bair-Merritt. 2016. Household and community-level adverse childhood experiences and adult health outcomes in a diverse urban population. *Child Abuse and Neglect* 52:135–145.

Welch, L. C., J. M. Teno, and V. Mor. 2005. End-of-life care in black and white: Race matters for medical care of dying patients and their families. *Journal of the American Geriatrics Society* 53(7):1145–1153.

Wright, A. A., B. Zhang, A. Ray, J. W. Mack, E. Trice, T. Balboni, S. L. Mitchell, V. A. Jackson, S. D. Block, P. K. Maciejewski, and H. G. Prigerson. 2008. Associations between end-of-life discussions, patient mental health, medical care near death, and caregiver bereavement adjustment. *JAMA* 300(14):1665–1673.

Appendix A

Statement of Task

An ad hoc committee will plan and host a 1-day workshop whose agenda will examine access to and equity of care for people with serious illness. The workshop will feature invited presentations and panel discussions on topics that may include

- Barriers that impede access to care for serious illness (e.g., advance care planning, palliative care, and hospice) among vulnerable populations and strategies to address those barriers;
- Strategies to build trust and effectively engage patients, families, and caregivers in diverse cultural, ethnic, racial, and socioeconomic environments, in order to communicate with patients and families in a culturally competent manner regarding expectations and values related to end-of-life care and to ensure that treatment is aligned with preferences;
- Approaches to enhancing the diversity of the workforce providing care to people with serious illness;
- Models of care delivery that currently serve vulnerable populations with serious illness, including public–private partnerships and community-level interventions, such as use of community health coaches for peer-to-peer interventions and partnering with faith-based organizations; and
- Research gaps and key questions for further research.

The planning committee will develop the agenda for the workshop, select speakers and discussants, and moderate the discussions. A proceedings of the presentations and discussions at the workshop will be prepared by a designated rapporteur in accordance with institutional guidelines.

Appendix B

Workshop Agenda

8:00 am   **Registration and Breakfast**

8:30 am   **Welcome from the Roundtable on Quality Care for People with Serious Illness**

Leonard D. Schaeffer, University of Southern California (*Chair*)

James Tulsky, M.D., Harvard Medical School, Brigham and Women's Hospital, and Dana-Farber Cancer Institute (*Vice Chair*)

Overview of the Workshop

Darci Graves, M.P.P., M.A., Special Assistant to the Director, Centers for Medicare & Medicaid Services

Peggy Maguire, J.D., President, Cambia Health Foundation

Workshop Planning Committee Co-Chairs

8:45 am   **Session 1**

Overview of the Landscape for Improving Access to and Equity of Care for People with Serious Illness

Moderator: Peggy Maguire, J.D., President, Cambia Health Foundation

- Bridgette Hempstead, President and Founder, Cierra Sisters
- Marshall Chin, M.D., M.P.H., Richard Parrillo Family Professor of Healthcare Ethics, Department of Medicine, The University of Chicago Medicine
- Kimberly Sherell Johnson, M.D., Associate Professor of Medicine, Senior Fellow in the Center for the Study of Aging and Human Development, Duke University School of Medicine
- Edward Machtinger, M.D., Professor of Medicine, Director, Center to Advance Trauma-informed Health Care and Director, Women's HIV Program, University of California, San Francisco

Panel Discussion/Audience Q&A

10:15 am   **Break**

10:30 am   **Session 2**

Improving Access to Care and Achieving Health Equity for People with Serious Illness: Organizational and Community Perspectives

Moderator: Nadine Barrett, Ph.D., M.A., M.S., Assistant Professor, Department of Community and Family Medicine, Duke School of Medicine

- Sister Anne Francioni, RN, M.A., SSND, Executive Director, Whole Kids Outreach

- Adán Merecias, Community Health Worker, Patient Navigator Program Manager, Familias en Acción
- Sandy Chen Stokes, RN, M.S.N., Founder, Chinese American Coalition for Compassionate Care

Panel Discussion/Audience Q&A

12:00 pm   **Lunch**

1:00 pm   **Session 3**

Improving Access to Care and Achieving Health Equity for People with Serious Illness: Patients/ Families and Clinicians

Moderator: Darci Graves, M.P.P., M.A., Special Assistant to the Director, Centers for Medicare & Medicaid Services

- Video: *Jay: Privilege and Discrimination in One Man's Life*
- Alice Huan-mei Chen, M.D., M.P.H., Deputy Director and Chief Medical Officer, San Francisco Health Network, Professor of Clinical Medicine, Department of Medicine, University of California, San Francisco
- Justin J. Sanders, M.D., M.Sc., Faculty, Serious Illness Care Program, Ariadne Labs, Attending Physician, Psychosocial Oncology and Palliative Care Department, Dana-Farber Cancer Institute and Brigham and Women's Hospital, Instructor in Medicine, Harvard Medical School
- Liz Margolies, LCSW, Founder and Executive Director, National LGBT Cancer Network

Panel Discussion/Audience Q&A

2:30 pm   **Break**

2:45 pm   **Session 4**

A Policy Agenda to Improve Access to Care and Achieve Health Equity for People with Serious Illness

Moderator: Sarah Downer, J.D., Associate Director, Whole Person Care and Clinical Instructor on Law, Health Law and Policy Clinic, Harvard Law School

- Diane Rowland, Sc.D., Executive Vice President, Henry J. Kaiser Family Foundation
- Andy Slavitt, M.B.A., Founder and General Partner, Town Hall Ventures, Former Acting Administrator, Centers for Medicare & Medicaid Services
- Lori Bishop, M.H.A., B.S.N., RN, CHPN, Vice President of Palliative and Advanced Care, National Hospice and Palliative Care Organization

Panel Discussion/Audience Q&A

4:00 pm   **Session 5**

Next Steps for Implementing Solutions to Improve Access to Care and Achieve Health Equity for People with Serious Illness

Moderator: Shonta Chambers, M.S.W., Executive Vice President, Health Equity Initiatives and Community Engagement, Patient Advocate Foundation

- Daniel Dawes, J.D., Director of the Satcher Health Leadership Institute, Morehouse School of Medicine, Principal Investigator and Co-Founder, Health Equity Leadership & Exchange Network

- Steven Clauser, Ph.D., M.P.A., Director, Healthcare Delivery and Disparities Research Program, Patient-Centered Outcomes Research Institute
- Nadine Barrett, Ph.D., M.A., M.S., Assistant Professor, Department of Family and Community Health, Duke University School of Medicine
- Peggy Maguire, J.D., President, Cambia Health Foundation

Panel Discussion/Audience Q&A

5:25 pm   **Closing Remarks**

5:30 pm   **Adjourn**